THE MEDICINE WOMAN

THE MEDICINE WOMAN
A Path of Power and Healing with Love and Plants

Linda Bates

AEON

First published in 2025 by
Aeon Books

Copyright © 2025 by Linda Bates

The right of Linda Bates to be identified as the author of this work has been asserted in accordance with §§ 77 and 78 of the Copyright Design and Patents Act 1988.

All rights reserved. No part of this publication may be reproduced, stored in a retrieval system, or transmitted, in any form or by any means, electronic, mechanical, photocopying, recording, or otherwise, without the prior written permission of the publisher.

British Library Cataloguing in Publication Data

A C.I.P. for this book is available from the British Library

ISBN-13: 978-1-80152-172-7

Typeset by Medlar Publishing Solutions Pvt Ltd, India

www.aeonbooks.co.uk

DEDICATION

This book is dedicated to:

Plants and their healing force/vitality

Linda's patients

Believers and users of plant-based medicines

Sifu Joshua Smith (Linda's son)

Salona Shresthra (Linda's daughter-in-law)

Aadiya Smith (Linda's granddaughter)

CONTENTS

FOREWORD — xi

PREFACE — xv

INTRODUCTION — xvii

SECTION ONE—THE VILLAGE HERBALIST

CHAPTER ONE
Finding my path — 3

CHAPTER TWO
Becoming the village herbalist — 11

CHAPTER THREE
My garden pharmacy — 21

CHAPTER FOUR
Two weeks in intensive care—Tom's story — 25

CHAPTER FIVE
A vicious assault—Andrew's story   39

CHAPTER SIX
Herbs and hearts—Ruby's story   43

CHAPTER SEVEN
Can you save my leg?—Klaus's story   47

CHAPTER EIGHT
No more surgery needed—Anita's story   51

CHAPTER NINE
The doctor's husband   61

CHAPTER TEN
My brain is eating my pituitary gland—Karen's story   65

SECTION TWO—FINDING THE SHAMAN

CHAPTER ELEVEN
The earth called me   73

CHAPTER TWELVE
Findhorn and shamanic work   77

CHAPTER THIRTEEN
Travelling to Findhorn   79

CHAPTER FOURTEEN
The train to Scotland   85

CHAPTER FIFTEEN
The Original Quest with Franco Santoro   89

CHAPTER SIXTEEN
Flowers: a gift of love from the earth   95

CHAPTER SEVENTEEN
Memories in the land   101

CHAPTER EIGHTEEN
My Chamomile and Lavender cloak   105

SECTION THREE—THE ART OF PRESCRIBING, MIXING, AND DOSING WITH HERBAL TINCTURES

CHAPTER NINETEEN
How to start   109

CHAPTER TWENTY
In the consultation room   115

CHAPTER TWENTY ONE
The importance of manufacturing processes   123

CHAPTER TWENTY TWO
Who tells you what doses to use?   127

CHAPTER TWENTY THREE
The influence of the *British Herbal Pharmacopoeia*   131

CHAPTER TWENTY FOUR
Case studies   137

CHAPTER TWENTY FIVE
Topical applications   163

BIBLIOGRAPHY   173

RESOURCES   175

FOREWORD

By Sonya Byron, Dr Sue Evans and Dr Ses Salmond

Linda Bates—the person

Linda Bates was a true healer and village herbalist in every sense of the word. She had a profound love and an unrivalled knowledge of the power of plant medicine, and the majority of the herbal remedies and flower essences she used in her 40 years of clinical practice, she grew and manufactured herself.

She was at least a fourth-generation herbalist, descended from a long line of gypsy healers, wise women, wild gatherers, and wildcrafters of herbal medicines. To Linda, every plant had an energetic healing property as well as medicinal quality. Infused into every part of her being was a true connection with and love of plants; she lived, breathed, and communicated with plants every day of her life. Her favourite herbs were Lavender, Angelica, Dandelion, Rosemary, and St John's wort.

Linda was a wise herbal Elder, a gifted and generous teacher and mentor, compassionate and passionate about sharing her love and knowledge of herbal medicine. She made an enormous contribution to teaching the art of making plant medicines sustainably and ethically and she was highly regarded within her profession. She was awarded life membership of the Naturopaths and Herbalists Association of

Australia in 2023, in recognition of her outstanding contribution to herbal medicine.

She was loved by so many, with family and friends, colleagues, students, and clients all over the world. She spent time living in Findhorn, a spiritual community in Scotland that recognises the intelligence of plants, where she created a beautiful healing garden that was in harmony with nature.

In addition to her herbal lineage, Linda studied with Dorothy Hall and Dennis Stewart, two leading herbalists in Australia in the 1980s. This gave her a deeply nuanced understanding not only of the herbs themselves but of dosing, vitality, temperament and of allowing the plants to do their magic to heal every ailment.

She was unapologetically herself and bravely and courageously spoke on behalf of the plants and of traditional herbal medicine practice.

Sadly, Linda died on 12 September 2024 before this book that she was so proud of was published.

The book—The Medicine Woman: A Path of Power and Healing with Love and Plants *by Linda Bates*

This book is Linda Bates's parting gift of generosity, of the healing power of plants and the humble learnings that she gained from each of the patients that feature in her case studies. Linda always let the herbs do the talking and was courageous in the cases she took on and fierce in her defence of the plants and her patients' well-being. The results often seemed miraculous as described in the following pages.

Linda connected with and inspired her herbal colleagues to adopt a more plant-centred approach to practice. According to Linda, plants are our birthright and traditional herbal medicine uses the vitality of the plant to restore the vitality of the patient. In other words, the life force in the plant heals the life force in the patient.

Linda believed in the power of the simplicity of the plants and in the simplicity of the connection between plant, healer, and patient. Her unique strengths were her extensive clinical experience, her ability to deeply engage with the story of each patient, her recognition of the miraculous healing power of plants, and her ability to make her own herbal medicines in service of her patients by hand, infused with her love and her magic.

The herbs were always with Linda and she made a lasting impression on her thousands of patients, in some cases seeing four generations of the same family. The plants never let her down and the case histories in her book attest to this.

Linda's legacy is her passion for herbs and herbal medicine. She was proud to call herself a herbalist, and she reminded us all of the grassroots nature of herbal medicine and how important it is to stay connected to our traditional roots and the philosophy of herbal medicine.

She will always be remembered as a lovingly fierce, staunch and vocal advocate for all things plant-based. Through her gift of this book, Linda invites you now on a magical journey of the healing power of plants.

PREFACE

All my life herbs have been my friends. Wherever I am in the world I can find wild herbs to heal and support me. When I am overwhelmed with grief and cannot eat, they rebuild me. When I have a serious infection they restore my immunity, clean out the invaders, and give me the strength and will to rebuild my health. When my heart is broken I sit with them and feel held in their aura of love. I can drink the morning dew from their flowers and find emotional support.

Since 1984 I have been a herbalist with a busy clinic and a teacher with apprentices and students. Herbs, whole, and harvested with their flowers, heal living things on all levels—emotional, spiritual, physical, functional, electrical, and structural. They are the only things found to contain the ingredients known to repair, restore, and rebuild human tissue, organ function, and body systems. These ingredients are understood to be medicinally active. Modern research has done much to present in scientific terms what traditional healers have always known: herbs are effective.

Herbs give us life and support us to live.

They are so powerful that since 1500 BC our world has gone through a long history of: respecting and worshipping them along with the medicine women and men who use them with skill; being fearful of the power of the medicines and the healers; rejecting them, banning them, and, at the command of the Christian church, burning the healers for working against the power of God. The arrests, tortures, and burnings went on for 400 years across England and Europe. During this time the lands and homes of the healers were confiscated and the Earth religion of the people was wiped out.

After the healers were stripped of their role in communities and society, the rich and powerful men of Europe began developing a branch of medicine intended to make a fortune from imitating the active ingredients contained in the plants.

Regardless of all of this terrible history, our herbs continue to grow and to heal. People continue to use them and to pass on knowledge about how to utilise them. According to the World Health Organisation (WHO), 75 per cent of the world's population uses their own traditional herbal medicine. This is not only because they cannot afford pharmaceutical medicine, or it's not available, but because they know it works and they respect their local healers.

The food of an area and the local people's traditional medicine is known to be of cultural and spiritual significance. The power of medicinal herbs can no longer be denied. In my opinion, people would be better served by going to a local traditional herbalist as their first port of call.

More recently in Australia and Europe we are developing a manufacturing industry with research and science, education and legislation. This industry is making herbs into herbal tablets, capsules, tinctures, and blends. Doctors are now being trained on how to use these tablets and capsules—often containing just one standardised herb at a time. This is not traditional herbal medicine.

Even amongst those who practise herbalism there can sometimes be confusion as to how to create blends for individual patients and what doses of herbal tinctures are to be used to create effective long-term repair. This book draws on my extensive experience to guide and support those stepping out onto the path of herbal healing with deep understanding, confidence, heart, and love.

INTRODUCTION

I grew up in England and Greece in the 1950s and 1960s. My understanding of what herbal medicine can do in the body comes from growing up using fresh plants as strong infusions, or just picking the leaves and eating them. I was attuned from quite young to feeling those herbs acting fast in my body—straight from the wild hedgerows and fields. No one was cultivating them in vast paddocks or coaxing them along in a backyard.

Those plants grew up in earth that was enriched year after year by hundreds of plants dying down into the soil for winter; with wild animals, farmed animals, and birds roaming the land, all the time adding their faeces and their lives back into the earth—fertilising and spreading seeds all over the planet.

In the 1950s and 1960s in England, pharmacists were also trained to make and use herbal tinctures. The introduction of pharmaceutical products and pharmaceutical medicine was in its early days and believe it or not the chemists were still being taught to use herbs and how to mix them for their customers. As they had done throughout time, the people came to report their ailments and wait while first the apothecaries and then the pharmacists mixed up herbs for them out the back. They always had a backroom full of tinctures and they often worked out what we needed over the counter without a doctor's prescription. When we needed medicines we went with mum and she knew what to ask for. We enjoyed the discussion with the chemist. If dad was away, we went walking to see what we could find to make our own medicines. We knew the fresh plants were better.

In my family, the doctor was not often consulted. When visited he would look at your tongue and the back of your throat, listen to your heart and breathing with his stethoscope, look in your ears using a magnifying instrument, and sometimes look in your eyes with another special tool. He would closely examine your eyes, including under the eyelids, with an iriscope light, and seriously consider whether you needed a few days in bed with light food and hot Ginger, Lemon and Honey drinks, or a herb mix for coughs and colds from the local chemist. If you showed signs of a fever alongside the sore throat, cough, and head congestion, he might consider a course of antibiotics. Very occasionally he would arrive for a home visit with his black bag full of the examining instruments. Mostly he would prescribe bed rest and extra special care from mum.

The women in my family shared their opinions of modern medicine, just between ourselves. My great-grandmother and grandmother said that modern drugs were a giant experiment on the human race and they were to be avoided at all costs. Herbs could be depended upon to work consistently without poisoning us. But they said softly, 'Don't tell too many people that we use herbs when we are sick because we might get into trouble'.

In 1957 we went to live in Cyprus for nearly four years. We lived in Limassol with the Greek people. No cars and no doctors. Plenty of herb medicine though and plenty of Greek people to help us with any herbs we might need for treating ourselves.

Then it was back to England. The 1960s was the era in which we all discovered what the drug Thalidomide can do to human beings. We weren't impressed. Antibiotics impressed everyone though: for a very long time so many people had died from pneumonia, scarlet fever, meningitis, sepsis, TB, diphtheria, influenza, and whooping cough. These infections were frightening to everyone, but antibiotics all but eliminated that fear.

The wounded soldiers during World War I mostly died from their infected wounds. The use of antibiotics started in the late 1930s to successfully treat all these life-threatening illnesses and they gave us hope and a belief that science was on the right path. We all began to believe in the miracles of science and medicine. My family continued to use herbs we collected in the wild ourselves and talk to the pharmacist over the counter for a mix of tinctures.

Antibiotics and the early vaccinations against polio, tetanus, smallpox, TB, and cholera helped everyone believe modern pharmacy would continue to make miracles happen. At last the future of modern medicine was hopeful for everyone. Not for me though. My body wasn't happy on antibiotics. I still used herbs.

In the 1990s, while working in the upper Blue Mountains of New South Wales (NSW) in Australia, I was told by some of my elderly patients, who had grown up in small Outback towns, that in the 1950s and 1960s in these towns there were no doctors. In their towns, the Chinese grocery shops had a Chinese herbalist out the back. They told me they were taken to the shop for help from the herbalist when they were sick. I had many patients then who were in their 80s and very happy to welcome me to the community. The ones who grew up in Sydney were familiar with going to a pharmacy for herbs mixed up on the spot by the pharmacists who in those days were still being trained to make and use herbal tinctures.

I arrived with my family in Adelaide in 1966. I went looking for the herbs I needed and found them at the central market with the Greek people. Those supplies of culinary herbs from the Greek growers were my lifeline. The early organics market in Australia had a big following in Adelaide. So I had access to pure, whole food and digestive help with European herbs.

In Sydney, Australia, in the late 1970s, I began my formal studies with Denis Stewart and then Dorothy Hall. The herbal medicines that were available for us to use then were manufactured by Nature Spirit and all their tinctures were 1:8 and almost clear—like water—and tasted more like ethanol alcohol than a herb.

At that point Dorothy Hall had 30 years of experience in prescribing and formulating herbal mixes for individual patients, and I have never, to this day, come across a patient who could say that she failed in her treatments. People who talk to me about being treated by Dorothy always smile wistfully and tell me nostalgically, 'Dorothy's herbs healed me'. So the highest compliment from one of these ex-patients of Dorothy's has been for them to say that I have 'fixed' them and then to add, 'Thank goodness I found you'.

The practitioners who studied with Dorothy use herbs as their first line of treatment: they use herbal medicines with knowledge and confidence. Dorothy Hall is remembered with love and gratitude by all those who have been treated by her and all those who have been taught by her.

She taught us to formulate for the individual, after the consultation, with five herb tinctures in a mix of 100 ml. And to dose at approximately 25 drops three times daily—this is approximately 1 ml each dose and adds up to 3 ml per day, or 21 ml per week. For each of the five herb tinctures in this mix, this is a weekly dose of 4.24 ml. She also taught us that this daily dose was only for chronic conditions.

The idea of drop dosing being effective is ridiculed by some who claim that drop dosing is not therapeutic or physical. To the practitioners of traditional herbal medicine the idea that drop dosing does not have therapeutic effects is ridiculous. It is a well-acknowledged traditional practice in Western Herbal Medicine. So is the use of fresh plant tinctures or infusions.

The third section of this book, the 'how to' section, is intended to show you that dosing is a creative art and that your ability to prescribe effective dosing will improve with experience and guidance from an experienced traditional herbalist. How to dose is as confusing as how to mix and what to mix, and all decisions about the mix and the dosing strategy you choose will be guided by the following:

1. Which herbs are in your mix? Are they gentle-acting mild herbs or are they medium-strength herbs? Are they very active strong herbs, many of which are only intended for short-term use? Are they mixed well—with the best considerations of supporting the best repair and the most gentle, balancing, and harmonising actions in the body? Are your dose recommendations gentle enough or too heroic and risky? Will your mix be restoring your patient's body with kindness?
2. The patient and the ground of illness—their life circumstances, their health or illness history, their strength, the intensity and severity of their symptoms, whether the condition is chronic or acute, how long they have had these symptoms (consider here the condition of chronic fatigue with its cycles of severity and improvement), and the current demands on their energy and time.
3. Whether you will be using tinctures or infusions and whether you are using dried herb material or fresh plant. Whether your tinctures

have been manufactured by the method of traditional maceration or the modern pharmaceutical method of percolation.
4. Where the plant material has come from, where it was grown, how it was grown, how it was harvested, how it was dried and how old it is.

Throughout this book, I use capital letters for the name of each herb. To me, they are real individual energies—full of life force. They are real characters in my world, ready to help and support us, waiting to hold our hands and restore us. As I re-read these case studies I am amazed at the actual healing power of these herbs, my friends.

The incredible tragedy is that we have allowed ourselves to be separated from our medicine women, who would have supported us throughout life. We have allowed ourselves to be seduced and mesmerised by the marketing skills of the pharmaceutical industry. And to listen to the ignorant who say, 'There is no evidence of efficacy' or 'Herbs are dangerous'.

Diet and long-term treatments

I haven't documented here any dietary recommendations for the patients (apart from a couple). In my practice, I always supervised and supported dietary changes which could lead them to healthier choices and easier-to-digest food combining in their meals to support long-term health improvements.

SECTION ONE

THE VILLAGE HERBALIST

CHAPTER ONE

Finding my path

I found magic in the earth from a very early age and in my relationships with plants with what they gave to me. I discovered that the earth could fill me with energy if my feet were bare, and that I could use this energy to fill myself and expand my heart. All this magic I wanted to share.

The organisers of the first Australian Naturopathic Summit in 2017 asked me to give a talk about my life and my path as a herbalist. They wanted to know what made me choose to be a herbalist and to hear some of the highlights that kept me on the path and made it so heartwarmingly satisfying.

I dug down deep into my Self, my child self, my young self, and my adult self. I gathered up the evidence in the family stories and my memories about the events and the people on the outside of my Self that seemed to help me make sense of this path. As I did my research I realised that my fate was probably written in the stars and that choice had very little to do with it. That is what my mother had told me. She said, 'You have choices but …'

When I was young I thought I had a choice about which turn to take at any time. Looking back I see that many times I had no choice. For me it was all about love. It was the path of my heart's journey into love, connection, and participating in community. I became a herbalist because it was my way to become valued and to contribute to people's lives.

I learned quite young that I could also draw down white light from the heavens, bring it in through the top of my head and into my heart, and then allow it to flow out through my arms and into others. This made me feel useful and connected. I thought my heart could become strong enough to bring magic into other people's hearts and hoped that this would open them to the earth and to each other.

My great-grandmother was a Romany gypsy herbalist. I come from a family of women who believed that periodically a herbalist would be born into the family, bringing with her the knowledge and wisdom from past lives. Training with a skilful medicine woman awakens this knowledge. This belief came through the generations of women in my mother's line.

My nanna was the chosen one of the ten children in her generation, but she refused to inherit the role from her mother. She was frightened by a law that threatened healers. Living through two World Wars turned her into a survivor, running pubs and clubs, and performing song and dance to entertain the customers. She had four daughters and her mother, the gypsy herbalist, lived with them. The house was always full of people coming for help from the herbs, and words and healing hands of the women.

My mother was her grandmother's helper—picking herbs with her and listening and learning. My mother was beautiful and had a special loving soul. She was swept away by a handsome man in the Royal Air Force. I was born in 1950 at Changi Hospital, in Singapore. I lived there, near the walls of Changi prison in the post-war celebratory atmosphere of the British colonial administration, with Chinese servants and Chinese herbs until I was about three.

Apparently, I was an absconder, dashing across the street into the jungle at every opportunity, throwing off my clothes on the way. Mum and the Chinese amah trained a dog to sniff me out and lead them to me. The trail of clothes gave them a good start. They often found me snuggling into the roots of big trees with green hands and bits of chewed-up plant matter dribbling down my chin. The Chinese amah was appointed by the RAF to help us at home and she was younger than my mum, who was still only 22. The amah used to take me to the kampong (village) in the jungle where her family lived so I could play with the children there. My dog came too and sometimes we stayed there with them for the night.

In 1953, when I was nearly 3 years old, I was taken to England on a big grey military ship all the way from Singapore. My dog had to stay there with my Chinese friends in the jungle. I cried. It was a long journey on that ship which was like a prison for me. And my life became memorable through the drama and the changes.

I arrived with my mum at her mother's house in the industrial town of Kettering in Northamptonshire. I was surrounded by dark red brick houses, row after row, and walls and back lanes and no front gardens. In the back gardens were the small cobbler's sheds and alleys into the back lanes so the night carts could come and collect the toilet waste from the cans in the outhouses. There, hanging on the wall, was a big tin bath ready for the weekly family bath time on Sundays in front of the fire in the kitchen.

I do clearly remember meeting my nanna, Kathleen, and her mother, Ruth, who still lived with them and was very old. My mother's three sisters were there and two cousins. The family story is that when I met my great-grandmother Ruth I tried to climb onto her knee. She stood up, took my hand and walked with me across the road and into the park which led to the river and into the woods.

My first walk into a wood in England is a strong visual memory. With my great-grandmother, the Romany gypsy herbalist, that's where I first met the magic trees of England and some of the herbs I would learn to work with. When we got back she sat down in her chair and announced to the women, 'This is the child with the gift and the love of the plants. I want to teach her everything I can. Brenda [Linda's mother], you have to help me. I don't have much time'.

The sisters were all astonished because we had been out for hours and my great-grandmother hardly ever walked very far. I remember her eating herbs along the way and helping me taste them and feel what they did to me. My memory of that walk is of the smells and tastes and feelings inside me and the visuals. She only lived a few more months but I did get a couple more walks. I remember my visits to her bedside, hopping into bed beside her, and watching everyone be sent away for a while.

My dad was scared to bits by all this since he was never quite sure whether he had married into a coven of witches … He spent a lot of time and energy trying to keep mum away from her family, and me well away from their influence. It didn't work. I loved them and I loved the woods across the road from my mother's family home in Kettering.

My father was away a lot, training to become a Canberra jet pilot with the Royal Air Force. Mum and I began a life of moving from place to place, boarding with people, to be close to dad so he could come home on weekends on his motorbike. I never knew anyone for long, and hardly ever met another child, so plants and animals were my companions. I continued to be an absconder, disappearing into the woods and bringing home plants to talk about and telling mum what the plants told me.

In my earliest memory of feeling the power of herbs, I was staying at my nanna's place. I was about 4 years old and had bronchitis. I was ordered to stay in bed under layers of eiderdowns. My nanna started brewing and mashing plant bits. My cousins warned me this wouldn't be nice and I should try to escape with them and hide at their place. But I was happy there so I stayed. My nanna pressed plants in her mortar and pestle and mixed the juices together with Lavender and Eucalyptus oil into some of her precious goose grease from the tin at the back of the larder. She stood me in front of the fire and slopped it all over my neck, back and front, down my chest and my upper back, around the sides of my face and under my nose.

Then she wrapped me in old torn sheets and popped me back under the eiderdowns with two hot water bottles. She brought me strong herbal infusions to drink, with a bit of brandy added. I swear I could feel those herbs going in through my skin, and down my throat, and helping me. I loved it. I sweated and coughed up lumps of mucus and was better in no time. I told my cousins it was wonderful, but they didn't believe me.

My mother tried not to talk too much about medicine and herbs because my father disapproved. Fortunately, he was away a lot and we always lived in the countryside, often in caravans, with woods and herbs all around.

I was 7 years old when we moved to Cyprus. Dad was an officer now and a qualified Canberra jet bomber pilot. We lived among the Greeks in Limassol and we had a Greek housekeeper. In 1957 the only people with cars on the island were the British Armed Forces, everyone else had donkeys and carts. I don't think there were any doctors there. Not many shops either. Just farmers markets, actually, with stalls, and Greek women selling their produce and advising on what herbs would help the family ailments. Long, easy exchanges over the weekly shopping and a Greek housekeeper to give us her traditional wisdom, cooking, and recipes.

I had a seriously sensitive digestive system—irritable bowel syndrome they call it these days—and multiple allergies, which meant I needed lots of help from the herbal world and lots of discussions about my body and my symptoms. My body has helped me learn a lot. I loved food and excelled at sport and gymnastics, so I was very strong. My favourite bag of lollies from the sweet shops in England was a bag of Liquorice sticks to chew all day.

Like a lot of RAF kids, I was sent off at the age of ten to a boarding school. It was in the north of England in an eighteenth-century mansion with a walled kitchen garden and a library full of old books. Rise Hall was the name of the mansion and it belonged to the Bethel family who had sensibly built a modern home on their property, and gone to live in it.

We were 45 kids with six rebellious-thinking nuns belonging to the Canonesses of Saint Augustine, a religious order dedicated to teaching young women and caring for the sick. These six nuns who ran our small school had broken away from the main branch of the order in the nearby city of Hull. They were dedicated to educating us girls differently. At weekends only five of us kids didn't go home and we were like a family. On weekends we ate together, went shopping in the local village each Saturday and grew lots of veggies and herbs in the walled kitchen garden.

One of the nuns knew about local and native medicinal herbs and how to use them. We shared long walks through the woods every weekend with her to spend our pocket money in the village. We also gardened together, so our conversations included sharing our knowledge of herbs and cooking, herbs and medicine. In spring I used to bring back medicinal herbs from the woods and plant them in the kitchen garden. We knew they weren't weeds and we made ourselves herbal infusions to help us with our colds, and other blends for my digestive difficulties.

At 16 years old, I was dragged, against my will, to Australia because the Australian Air Force bought my father's contract for his skills as a jet pilot to train their pilots and to lead upper atmosphere research teams in Australia. In 1966 my research into what Australia had to offer me wasn't reassuring. There was Skippy, but *no* Tamla Motown music, *no* Ban the Bomb marches, *no* Beatles or Rolling Stones concerts. I won't go on. I tried my best to get out of going.

When I got here it was even worse than I could have imagined. We went to Adelaide, the city of churches. No one had even heard of Mary Quant or mini skirts! Worst of all, mum and I couldn't find the herbs I needed regularly. I quickly learned to drive and wandered around until I found some herbs I recognised in the Adelaide Hills. Then I found the early organic movement and the bulk-buying shops, and the Adelaide Central Market with Greek and Italian stallholders selling their market garden produce and lots of herbs.

I was a lost soul really—the new girl yet again at my 14th school. I found no one I could relate to—just plants and the earth. My fascination with healing and managing the body made dad hope that I might become a doctor. His biggest dread was that I might be one of the witches of my mother's family.

However, since those women had passed down to me the idea that pharmaceutical companies were perpetrating a giant experiment on the human race, I already didn't have much respect for that path. I found an English Repertory Company and a small theatre with a youth group and a new interest with friends of all ages.

When I was ready for university I went to Flinders and enrolled in Drama, English, and Philosophy. My dad still hasn't forgiven me. He thinks I wasted my brain.

After university I had a wonderful ten-year career in stage and production management with opera, musical theatre, and dance companies in Adelaide, Sydney, and London. I carried bags of herbs and tissue salts to keep me going and for anyone else in need. I worked on the opening season of the Sydney Opera House and made herb teas for Joan Sutherland's sore throat. Those adventures are like another life for me—they gave me an extended family as well as a connection to creativity, teamwork, and caring for each other.

I collected books on herbs for healing all through those halcyon years of the 1970s and I found my teachers in Sydney in the late 1970s and early 1980s, Denis Stewart and then Dorothy Hall. While I worked with the pre-production team for the film *Mad Max 2* I went to a herbalist trained by Dorothy Hall for help with my digestive system. That was it for me. It felt like I became reconnected to my path. Dorothy Hall, teaching us from 30 years of clinical experience, spoke my language, and began to awaken in me the knowledge I brought with me into this life, according to the beliefs of my women's line. Managing my body became easy and my understanding of what healing is and what herbs can do expanded into something unique and extraordinary.

All my life people seem to be able to tell me their troubles. And I have always been convinced there is a solution or some support from the earth available, if they want to use it. It must come from my family background (maybe it is in my genes) and my experience of what plants have done to support me. I believe that plants have the power to heal us physically *and* change our emotional states—as flower essences do. Herbal medicines, made with fresh plants, capture the energy field and the vital force of the whole plant. Depending on where it is grown, the quality of the soil that the plant has grown in, the time of year it is picked, whether it is picked with love, and how it is handled during the making of medicine—all these factors give each medicine some variation in potential actions and strengths.

I started making my own creams for skincare in the early 1970s. My nanna showed me how to do it with the animal fats from roasting meats. The English call this fat 'lard'. I used this as my base cream and added the pressed juice from fresh herbs. The lard from roasted goose makes the best creams but was hard to get hold of! In later years I took to using lanolin—but I was never sure why the sticky fat from the fleece of a sheep would be soaked up by the skin of a human being. So I melted it down and beat in lots of organic vegetable and nut oils along with the herb juices. Then I gave up using the lanolin and replaced it in my recipes with raw beeswax from a nearby honey producer. My skin was really happy.

I believe that my skin creams provide the body with the very best way to absorb essential fatty acids and herbs. The good oils are taken in through the skin and go straight into the bloodstream. When herbs are also in the cream they are carried by those oils into the body and within 30 seconds they are available wherever needed. No stress on the liver or digestive system to carry the ingredients to where needed, and no chance of the herbs being used by another part of the body along the way.

CHAPTER TWO

Becoming the village herbalist

In 1992 I moved to Mount Victoria, in the Blue Mountains, with my 10-year-old son, Joshua, after a broken marriage. I bought an old cottage with a neglected garden and began to immediately gather and plant my European herbal allies. I wanted to have fresh plants available again to support my life force.

Joshua and I went to enrol him at the local primary school and we met with the school secretary who I later came to know as the Manager of Mount Victoria! While she and I talked, Josh loudly and proudly announced, 'My mum is a herbalist'. I winced.

I thought it was a bit soon to introduce my strange thinking into the school community. She turned to look out of the window with a glazed expression for what seemed like minutes. Slowly turning back to us she said, 'I dreamed that a herbalist was coming to help me through my menopause'.

This wonderful woman turned me into the village herbalist and brought me the clients. We'll call her Rose because she has no objection to me using her name and it feels respectful. First, she brought me her mum, Olive, who was in her 80s. Then she ordered a first aid kit for the school, asked the P&C (Parents and Citizens Association) to pay for it, as well as paying me to train her to use it. This started a string of orders from mums for first aid kits or herb creams to use at home. So I started making healing creams with fresh plant juices using the herbs in my garden. Making my medicine garden became my heart healing activity and I resumed my lifelong passionate relationship with people in need, the earth, and fresh medicinal herbs.

I hung up my shingle (a business sign) on the side of the house near the gate, 'Linda Bates, Herbal Medicine. Welcome to the Clinic. Please knock or phone … for an appointment'. I found a lovely large pot, put an old-fashioned medicinal Rose (*Rosa rugosa*) in it, and placed it by my clinic door and this became the place where people collected their herb mixes from, and left me their payments. Small gifts were left too with thank-you notes.

Unsatisfied with the dried plant herb tinctures I had been buying from Nature Spirit for my dispensary I began making my own tinctures from organically grown fresh herbs picked in my garden or found wild in the upper mountains. My Sydney clients had no trouble coming up to see me in Mount Victoria and they began telling me that my mixes were becoming more effective and noticeably more powerful. Olive, Rose's mum, started telling me about growing up with herb medicines from the chemists in Sydney or popping into Chinese grocery shops because they often had a herbalist out the back with their dried Chinese herbs ready to mix up for your problem. Olive started spreading the word amongst the older women at the CWA (Country Women's Association) and when I successfully treated the ulcers on her leg, my leg ulcer protocol began to be wanted by the older residents of the upper mountains.

This protocol involved using my creams along with my instructions to use old sheets torn up and boiled for use as bandages. These bandages would hold the cream on overnight, and be taken off in the morning to give the ulcerated skin some fresh air. Then the patient should give the leg some direct sunshine for 15 minutes before 11 am each day. This treatment began to undermine the monthly income of the Blackheath doctors and pharmacists.

The doctor's protocol was to automatically book the older leg ulcer patient in for an appointment every week for up to a year to change the dressing and send them on their way. No sunshine or fresh air ever touched these leg ulcers! The dressings had to be bought by the patient from the local pharmacy and given to the doctor every week. These lovely pensioners were paying up to $100 per month out of their pensions. That was a lot of money in 1993. So with a bag of freshly picked herbs to make their own infusions or a small bottle of a herb mix to improve circulation and a jar of herb cream I saved the Medicare budget, and the pensioners, lots of money. And the leg ulcers got better real fast.

Olive loved my herbs and slowly she weaned herself off her tablets from the doctor. She usually told the doctor before she told me. I didn't encourage her to stop taking them. She just decided for herself. 'Load of rubbish', she said, 'they make me feel ill anyway but the doctor has to be told so he can keep an eye on me, check my blood pressure and all that'.

I got very worried and told her she shouldn't do that without talking to me first, so I could get her ready with herbs and then she could talk to the doctor about wanting to come off her pharmaceuticals. So that's what we did. It caused a deal of irritation for her doctor because she insisted on coming off her tablets.

Olive had leg circulation problems, bunions, chilblains, kidney stones, one kidney, high blood pressure, and leg ulcers. She responded so well to my treatments that after only two years with herbal footbaths and very low doses of my herb mixes she had no leg ulcers, no chilblains, no aching legs, and no need for high blood pressure pills or Zyloprim. Her doctor stopped me in the street and gave me a good telling off, as have many doctors over the years. Occasionally an angry phone call would come.

One doctor in the mountains rang me after he found out I was treating a child with asthma who was also his patient. I assured him I was being responsible and insisting the child stay on his medication and carry the Ventolin at all times for emergencies. I explained to him that some of my herbs were really great for asthma—for the repair of lungs and restoring full function. He was shocked—he said that if herbalists could treat asthma it would take away a lot of his annual income. He never sent me anyone with asthma to treat even though the child patient we shared did recover functioning lungs and had no need to stay on daily pharmaceutical tablets. The child got used to carrying the Ventolin just in case. His mother was my patient and they began using herb mixes for respiratory infections, to prevent his lungs from becoming damaged again.

Another doctor began sending me all his women patients with difficult menopausal symptoms after his wife did a workshop with me and came to consult me for herbal help to stabilise her menopause difficulties. He became my doctor as I began to need a few check-ups and someone to keep an eye on my blood pressure. A few years later, when I went down very fast with what we later discovered was a dreadful lung infection caught from potting soil, this wonderful man abandoned his clinic for the day and came to me at home and saved my life.

He bundled me into his car and took me for X-rays, then to the pharmacy to collect immediate medication. He told the staff to get the X-rays ready for him as an emergency, took me home to bed, and told me to pack for the hospital. Two hours later he arrived back and told me the X-rays showed I had hardly any functioning lung space left to breathe and the infection was moving fast. He drove me straight to the emergency department at the local hospital. He packed my case as well because I was delirious and incapable. They saved my life, that doctor and the hospital.

He checked on me in hospital every couple of days. I got very close to death in my isolated room. My friends visited, with gowns and masks on, and brought me healthy liquefied foods full of herbs and special spring water. My close friend JD, a Chinese herbalist and acupuncturist, visited and left my body and ears covered in his strange acupuncture dots which mystified the nursing staff. And my beautiful son, Josh, came and sat by my bed to remind me of what I had to live for.

Ten days later my doctor arrived to sign me out and told me I would always have really scarred lungs after such a serious infection. I told him I wouldn't because I had herbs to repair my lungs. He didn't believe I could do that so we had a bet—$50 said I couldn't do it. I took my herbs and went for the X-ray after 12 months and we looked at it together. He congratulated me and paid me the $50 with amazement.

One Sunday morning JD rang to ask me to go with him and help another friend with Hodgkin lymphoma. She was suffering bad side effects from her latest chemotherapy treatment. He thought I could help with my fresh herbs. I wandered around my garden and collected a big basketful of gentle-acting, low-strength herbs as I held this woman in my energy field. (I had met her previously.) I collected him on the way and together we arrived at the woman's home.

While I gave her a Reiki treatment, JD chopped up all the fresh herbs and put them in my large enamel pot, added filtered water, and started the slow simmering process for an hour. We used a large amount of herbs in that mix. Together we helped her drink half a mugful every half hour for three hours. We were thrilled and amazed at how much strength and recovery those herbs gave her and so was she.

Frank was Rose's father-in-law. When he came to see me he was 89 and had painful joints, a shaky heart, and a very high PSA reading. He didn't want any doctor's drugs he told me. I gave him a 100 ml mix of seven herb tinctures, advised a very low dose (30 drops three times daily), and said we'd see how he did with them and adjust the dose if we had to. I always did that—started everyone on a low dose and checked in with them a week later to adjust the dose if the patient hadn't felt a noticeable difference in their symptoms. I believed the herbs could do as well as any doctor's drugs if I was clever enough with them. So I worked towards this always—keeping in touch with my patients to make sure.

Within a week Frank reported no pain in his joints and no shaky heart, and within a month his PSA reading was right down and he was a happy man. For years I delivered a repeat mix to Frank on my morning walk. He always invited me in for a morning cuppa and while we drank it by the kitchen wood stove he told me stories from his working life of driving trains around Outback NSW. Frank had 12 children and 50 grandchildren so you can imagine how his success story brought me a tidal wave of clients. He lived until he was 99 when his heart gave out. Apparently, he told the ambulance drivers and the Blue Mountains Hospital emergency staff: *If you would just get Linda Bates here, her herbs will bring me back and keep me going!* [More details about the herbs and dosages used in this story are detailed in Chapter 24, page 137.]

One morning Rose hammered on my back door and told me Olive had fallen down her back steps the previous evening and was a bit of a mess. Ten concrete steps. She didn't want to bother us until the morning. I grabbed the Arnica pillules, the Rescue Remedy, and a bottle of wildcrafted Hypericum flower-infused oil. I tipped a slug of Lavender essential oil into the Hypericum oil and ran up the hill with Rose towards Olive's house. Olive was black and blue all over and could hardly move. Her husband was yelling, 'She should go to hospital'. Olive was whispering and breathing very carefully. 'No way, what can they do? Linda will help me'.

Fortunately, she could walk if she had to and she was sure she had nothing broken. Barb helped me. We popped the first few Arnica pillules under her tongue and poured Edward Bach's Rescue Remedy all over her, very gently spreading it over her bruised areas. Then, still very gently, we spread the Hypericum oil, mixed with a little Lavender oil, over her bruises. Leaving Rose to repeat the same three treatments after an hour, I dashed off home to prepare some herb mixes—one of the fresh plant tinctures mixed into oils for adding to the bath and another for Olive to use internally. In four days there was no sign of the bruising and Olive was up and about happily telling everyone in town.

One day Rose's daughter, pregnant with twins, knocked on my door worried she was going to have a miscarriage. She was only just five months pregnant. A week later Rose rang me from Nepean Hospital to say that her daughter had been helicoptered down there and had given birth to her twins prematurely on arrival. Nine days later, it was Rose herself who was hammering on my door, shouting, 'Where are you? You gotta make us some herbs for the twins. You're our only hope. They just keep getting sicker'.

When I opened the door to Rose she was sobbing.

> *They can't breathe on their own, they've got tubes in, and now they are getting lung infections so they're being put on antibiotics, Ventolin, corticosteroids, and God knows what else. They can't keep their liquid formula food down, they're losing weight and going backwards. If you don't make us some herbs, those babies will die.*

I told her I'd never done such a thing. I didn't know how to dose such tiny babies. I knew the babies needed herbs every one to two hours. I told her that we couldn't expect the hospital staff to dose them and, in fact, we couldn't even tell the hospital staff what we were doing. The babies had to be given their herbs by Rose and her daughter every hour, day and night.

Rose told me they both understood all that and that they were ready to take turns at being there for those babies and to slip the herbs into their mouths when no one was looking. One of the babies had awful eczema and the other had asthma. So I mixed a slightly different mix for each baby and I removed the alcohol from both mixes. I mixed herbs to support their immunity and the growth and efficiency of their lungs and I told Rose to give them each 1 drop every hour, or as close to every hour as possible, and to ring me after 23 hours to report in. The report was good. So I increased the dose to 3 drops every hour. The next report was very good. Rose and her daughter were really onto the hospital staff and watching for whether those babies needed those drugs.

Since taking the herbs they had been keeping their food down and in five days they had taken the babies off the Ventolin and corticosteroids; in seven days they were off the antibiotics; in nine days the respirators were taken away. The hospital staff were mystified and impressed. Me too.

Those babies really thrived on herbs. They were home in no time and they took the same herb mixes constantly for almost three years. If they looked like getting a respiratory infection their mum gave them their herb mix for a few days and they got better. My notes tell me I made these mixes for them for five years. They are now in their early 20s. One has become a doctor and is adding Chinese herbal medicine to her skills. The other is a veterinary nurse. They have been high school athletics champions and high achievers. They are recorded as the only premature babies in Australia who have never had anything medically wrong with them or needed pharmaceutical medicine. [More details about the herbs and dosages used in this story are detailed in Chapter 24, page 137.]

There are many stories from these years. Some of the people who came to my door through my medicine garden recognised my plants, had some of them in their gardens, and asked me to teach them how to use plants as medicines. So I started groups of six people to meet once a month for a few hours in the morning. We would workshop the health issues of each person in the group, or a member of their family, while we drank herbal infusions. I taught them about the healing powers of three or four fresh herbs from my garden each time we came together. At the end of the morning, I sent them home with baby plants to put in their gardens or a bag of fresh herbs to make infusions for themselves.

These groups reconnected me to the power of fresh plants made into simple infusions. Some of these groups met for two years and in spring they often met every fortnight. In the first group, a woman with chronic thrush problems asked for help. She had been struggling with repetitive thrush for three years. My Calendula plants were flowering so we picked a bag of the flowers and I told her that for her treatments she was to take seven flowers and chop them up finely into a teapot. Then pour boiling water on them and leave them to steep for half an hour. After that pour the lot into a shallow bath and sit in it for half an hour while swishing the Calendula-filled water up into her vagina. I advised her to do this three times a week.

After four weeks she was to soak a sea sponge in good yoghurt and insert it into her vagina, leaving it for half an hour each day for a week. Five weeks of this treatment was enough. She had no return of the thrush for the two years we sat in class together. She went to live in Perth and used to let me know about every six months that she was still clear of the thrush. The great satisfaction for me is that she knows how to deal with it using a few flowers instead of taking something that costs too much and may poison her system. And that she would spread this knowledge to benefit women friends for the rest of her life.

In the Blue Mountains, I became a village herbalist. My clinic door was always welcoming. My heart was always full and strong. The people who came to my door made me into the medicine woman my great-grandmother saw in me. It was their needs, their trust and love that woke up the knowledge in me and made me such a strong part of their community.

The science, the research, and the development of manufacturers with quality products and their evidence of efficacy is so important. I love the fact that research using the methodology of modern science so often reassures us that what we've been using a plant for over hundreds of years is actually correct. This knowledge, passed down the centuries, is called empirical science. I am still using plants used and written about by Galen, a Greek physician, surgeon, and philosopher born in 130 AD whose medical research and findings have been used as the basis for the growth of knowledge in medicine for over 1,500 years; Avicenna, a Persian physician, born in 980 AD, who wrote *The Canon of Medicine*; and a woman known as Trotula of Salerno, who, in the twelfth century, wrote the earliest book in Europe on gynaecology and herbal medicine for women. This book is still used as one of the best medical treatises ever, and her work has been plagiarised by many.

Modern scientific research often gives us more—for example when it was discovered that *Hypericum perforatum* is also antiviral and works on lipid-enveloped viruses such as the very serious Epstein-Barr family of viruses, which includes chickenpox, herpes, shingles, and glandular fever. Add this to Hypericum's numerous uses throughout history for repairing the nerves, for pain relief, for depression, for detoxing the blood, and for restoring the liver, and we have a herb that will work in ways that nothing in modern pharmacy can match. However, processed *Hypericum perforatum* with a standardised amount of hypericin content can have undesirable side effects. I use very small doses and pick the wild fresh plant to make my medicines.

No matter how many pills or tinctures our manufacturers make with dried-up herb material and standardised levels of active ingredients, I still know with every cell of my being that the fresh ones work best; that some people still need to be taught that herbal medicine, in the hands of someone trained by an experienced clinician, can be miraculous; and that herbalists are not witches.

Herbalists are actually quantum scientists. They work with the love of the earth, the cycles of life, and the love of people. Herbs have kept my body strong, expanded my heart, and connected me to the hearts of others.

CHAPTER THREE

My garden pharmacy

It was a perfect spring day in the Blue Mountains. I was in my clinic making up the last herbal mix of the week for my patients. They would be collected on the weekend. This one was to repair the lungs and immunity of a 7-year-old boy who'd had asthma since he was a baby. His mother brought him to me two years previously. She didn't want him on the pharmaceutical drugs that made him feel so awful. He was wheezy all the time, couldn't run with his friends, and was often on antibiotics for bronchial infections. He was nauseous and anxious a lot, especially after using his Ventolin pump. He had started school as a sickly child and couldn't do sports.

Through the window I watched them walk past the house and head down through my medicine garden. The boy was skipping. Quickly I wrote his name on the label with dosage instructions and stuck the label on the bottle as the bell rang. I opened the door.

It was the boy holding out a bunch of flowers with a card he'd made at school. 'The flowers are for you. I made you the card 'cause you help me feel better'. He took a deep breath to show me he could. 'Mum said to tell you that I can run real fast now. Not many kids can beat me an' I hardly ever need my puffer'.

I squatted to receive his gift and handed him his bottle of herbs. 'Thanks. What a lovely card. I'm very happy that my herbs help you feel good, and I'm real proud to know such a fast runner. You just make sure you never forget to carry that puffer, just in case you need it. Where's mum?'

Before I could stand up he put his arms around my neck and hugged me tight, then pointed. 'She's sitting in the Lavender circle up there', he said. 'She's rubbing flowers and sniffing them. She likes it there'.

'Good. I'll walk up with you'.

We set off up the path and he slipped his hand into mine.

'Are any of your plants in my medicine?'

'They certainly are. Those Lavender flowers are in your medicine, and see this Ribwort here, you've got some of that too. The big bush over there with the golden leaves, outside the kitchen window, with white flower heads shaped like umbrellas—that's Elder and you have Elderberries in your mix, and this Peppermint—here smell this'.

I picked some Peppermint and rubbed it under his nose. He took it off me and popped it into his mouth, chewing happily.

'I know that one, that's real good. Mum said there's Ginger in my mix too?'

'There is. It's the Ginger that makes you feel all warm and relaxed deep inside. See that rosette of large, grey, hairy-looking leaves—that's Mullein and those leaves have helped you get better. Next time you come to pick up your herbs, those plants over there will be flowering. It's Echinacea. The flowers are glorious and they are in your special mix too'.

We reached his mum, still sniffing the Lavender flower squashed between her fingers.

'I've popped the money for the herbs in your pick-up pot by the back door. I'm gonna have to book him in for classes with you in a few years. He reckons he's gonna to be a herbalist. He wants to fix everyone's asthma. The doctor is a bit annoyed but what can you do? We're all real happy at home. He's a normal kid at last and loving his sport at school. Thanks. See you soon'.

I went in the back door for a herb tea. The golden Elder by the house coloured the light in my kitchen a warm yellow. In the morning the sun beams criss-crossed through the yellow making this corner feel blessed every day.

My Elder trees are my home guardians. I plant them around the fences and by the doors. Believed to be magical protectors, the spirits of these trees have been loved by generations of healers. Now modern science has discovered their flowers and berries are antiviral and antibacterial against a wide range of difficult respiratory infections. What an amazing time for me to be alive and a herbalist.

With my Chamomile and Lemon Verbena tea I went outside to relax on the Yarrow lawn among my herbal allies. If only my great-grandmother could see me now, or my grandmother, or my mother. I wondered if they'd had any premonitions, when they were teaching me, that one day I would be able to practice the traditional medicine so many generations of women had risked imprisonment, or their lives, for sharing.

My end-of-the-week peace was short-lived …

CHAPTER FOUR

Two weeks in intensive care — Tom's story

On the night of Friday 15 October 2003 one of my closest friend's son, Tom, aged 23, had a terrible motorbike accident on a dark country road in northern NSW. He was a wild, teasing, loving boy, and after an argument at home he drove off on his big powerful bike for a drink with his mates at the pub. A few hours and a few drinks later he challenged a mate to a race home, threw on his helmet without doing it up, and roared off. Two hundred metres from his home, and in the lead, he skidded on a corner, slid sideways through a fence, and lost his helmet just before slamming head-first into a tree. His friend skidded to a halt and ran towards Tom's body, picking up the helmet on the way.

He found Tom with blood pouring from his mouth. Fortunately, this friend had done a first aid course and so he put Tom in the recovery position and ran to the house to call an ambulance. The ambulance team did their best and Tom was still alive when they arrived at the hospital. His mother and father were called and they began their grieving.

At my home in the Blue Mountains I had finished my day of consultations in my clinic/studio, made up some herbal mixes to be collected in the morning, walked up to the house, had a cup of tea, cooked dinner, eaten, and put my feet up to watch a video. About 9 pm the phone rang. It was another friend telling me what had happened to Tom. The shock was gigantic. I was at Tom's birth. His family was my family. My son grew up with him. We spent our holidays and birthdays together. If they were sick, I made them herbal medicine, and they were mostly healthy.

I tried to phone Tom's mother and father, Marina and John. I couldn't find them. All I found out was that if he could be kept alive he would be air-lifted down to St George Hospital Intensive Care in Kogarah. I stayed up most of the night in shock using Rescue Remedy and Vital Spark to keep myself calm. I phoned my son Joshua, in Sydney, to ask him to find Tom's sister and stay with her while we all waited for news. They couldn't air-lift him until his condition was stable. I found a photograph of Marina, John, Tom, and his sister Sal. That night I sent Reiki to them all—often—and I designed what I would take to the hospital bedside to help bring Tom back. I finally fell asleep about 4 am.

At 7 am I was back in my clinic making herbal mixes to take to Tom's bedside. At 10 am I was still praying and mixing when Wendi Forbes called in to collect her medicines and to bring me presents—her set of healing oils: Heart Oil, Peace Oil, and Consecration Oil. She makes them while chanting Tibetan Buddhist mantras. She took one look at me. 'What on earth happened to you since I saw you yesterday? You look like you've been run over by a truck. I couldn't stop thinking about you all morning. That's why I've brought you my oils'. So I told her.

Wendi said to take the oils with me to the hospital and apply them to the family and friends—but first to myself right now—she showed me—applying Heart Oil to my crown chakra, third eye, throat, and heart chakras. My whole being sighed with relief. She told me, 'Apply Peace Oil and Consecration Oil to the palms of your hands before working on Tom, and breathe in the smell. Use all three oils on Tom every time you sit with him and make sure he can smell them'. Wendi left me preparing my medicines.

At about midday a friend called from Tom's family home. He told me that Tom was about to be air-lifted down to Sydney and Marina and John were being driven down by other friends. He said he felt sure Tom's spirit had left his body and wasn't going back. 'I believe that Tom's spirit will wait for us to repair his body before he returns to it', I replied.

I phoned my son, Josh, to let him know and arranged to meet him in Sydney. That Tom was still alive and being air-lifted gave me such relief that I fell asleep for a few hours.

I left home at 4 pm with a large cardboard box full of treatment options. I drove into Sydney, collected Josh, and arrived at the St George Emergency Care Unit at 6:30 pm. I was taken to a special room for the family with a kitchen, comfy chairs, table, dining chairs, a fridge, and two sofa beds. The paralysed shock in the room was intense. Tom's father, John, welcomed us with a hug, the others with their eyes.

My dear friend Marina, Tom's mother, looked shocking. Her skin was ghostly white, her body was rigid, and she could hardly speak. I knew if I hugged her she would fall apart. Alice, Tom's partner, was making tea. Gordon and his daughter Zoe were there. Zoe had grown up with Josh, Tom, and Sal. Gordon had driven John, Marina, Zoe, and Alice down to Sydney. Sal had arrived with a Sydney friend. No one had seen Tom or had any news.

I got out the Rescue Remedy, Vital Spark, and Heart Oil. I started giving it to Marina and asked, 'Would anyone else like some?' Someone said, 'I think we all want anything you've got for us'. We passed around the Rescue Remedy and Vital Spark while I demonstrated what to do with the Heart Oil. Someone else said, 'We'd like you to do it for us'. They all opened their shirts and waited. I applied Heart Oil to each of them in turn. They all visibly relaxed and the blood began to colour their faces. Some tears were released.

Tom was being operated on. His neck was broken in three places. He had five broken ribs, three of them puncturing his lungs, a mashed right shoulder, a left leg shattered with bits of bone sticking out in all directions, a skull and face that were cracked into many segments, and very severe brain damage. The surgery was to reset and pin together the leg and the shoulder, reset and brace the neck, and pull the ribs out of the lungs. The broken sections of his skull were hanging in the right place but separated by gaps because of severe swelling.

When one of the emergency care surgeon/specialists came to find us, he wanted a word with the parents. They asked for me to be present, said I was the mother's sister; it was the truth of how we felt. We were told that Tom was expected to die; that his injuries were so severe that it could be many months before he came out of coma, if ever, and the team all considered it impossible for him to recover. He said that the best outcome would be that Tom would be badly brain-damaged and advised us to prepare ourselves to let him go. Then they invited us in to see him.

Tom's father couldn't face going in yet. I had to go in—the sooner I could use flower essences, homoeopathy, herbs, and oils on Tom the better his chance of healthy recovery. I went in with Marina,

Tom's mother. Tom was unrecognisable. Apart from the extensive damage to his body and the wounds and swelling, he had tubes in his throat, his arms, his mouth, his lungs. He had a neck brace on, pins sticking out of his right shoulder, a cast on his left leg from the knee down, and a head probably three times normal size. We looked at each other and we knew we had to replace our shock, distress and anxiety with positive, loving, supportive energy. It was hard to repress the grief.

We asked Tom's nurse if we could apply some oils to his body and we began our work on him together. First we applied Rescue Remedy and Vital Spark all over him. Heart Oil, Peace Oil, Consecration Oil on the chakras. Then we covered him with my mixes of herbs and oils with homoeopathics added. The nurse sat at the end of his bed monitoring all his vital functions, medications, and machinery, and watched us, fascinated. He even let us saturate dressings with our preparations. We whispered loving words to Tom as we worked and we called him back to help us heal him. I surrounded him with Reiki symbols and poured my mixes gently and generously all over his battered head.

Only two visitors at a time, they told us. After an hour Marina left me there working on him. She told them all there in the family room that before they visit Tom's bedside they must clear their energy fields of all negativity and distress. Alice came in next and struggled with her emotions, just as they all did; then, one by one, Tom's close extended family—all wanting to hope and all praying to be effective in their support of his recovery.

As I sat next to his right ear giving him Reiki, I remembered conversations with my hypnotherapist friend about talking to the unconscious and the subconscious. My knowledge of anatomy and physiology helped me use this idea to calmly talk Tom through how he could help his brain to clear the leaked blood and fluid filling the damaged tissues, to heal the bruising in his brain. I spoke to his cellular activity. I used this idea every time I sat with Tom during his coma. I told him how to take my herbs and oils in through his skin and then through parts of his system to the injured areas. I talked as if we were in his body together. I described how it looked and felt as we moved around using the herbs and oils to mop up the mess.

By this time a spiritual healer in China and another in Queensland had been contacted and both were working with his spirit. Also, word had spread and later we worked out that about 100 people were focused on sending Reiki regularly. Two or three times a day I would phone a friend in the Nambucca Valley with news of Tom's progress and she would distribute it.

After a while, the staff asked us to leave him for the night. We gathered in the family room and held hands and prayed. Then we ate the meal someone had gone out to find and drank the wine and cried and talked about Tom's recovery, and I told them stories of what my herb mixes had done for people over the years. Marina and I went for a walk and she told me she didn't want Tom back with brain damage and neither did John.

She was very shaky and trying hard to be sensible. Marina is normally the capable rock that holds everyone else together, and organises them. In 26 years of friendship she has always arrived to care for me— through my two divorces, a nervous collapse, a partner's very serious accident, and me nearly dying of pneumonia. We had our babies together and when I needed a rest from my busy life I would have it on her veranda in the protective peace of her and John's home, while the kids played.

In our family room that first night we were restless and nervous and our naps were full of waking and walking the corridors. Convinced that our presence beside his bed was the best way to help Tom, we began ringing the bell early the next day to be let in to his bedside. The first sight of him that day was extraordinary. His swollen head was half the size and he was recognisable. The bruising was emerging, some was already yellow. Some of the nurses were impressed and stopped by briefly to talk. His personal nurse was enthusiastic. I told them it was a few herbs mixed with oils. They could smell the Lavender oil and talked of aromatherapy, massage, and Reiki. No one knew I was a herbalist.

By the end of the second day, the staff had given up asking us to leave so Tom could rest. They could feel we were peaceful and even their machines were telling them that Tom was benefitting from our concentrated presence. Even so only two at a time could stay by him. About every three hours I would repeat my routine, working on Tom for about half an hour.

On the second night, I was alone with Tom for a while applying the oils and talking to him. I couldn't resist putting 5 drops of Rescue Remedy and Vital Spark on his lips, alongside the breathing tubes. Then I put 5 drops of homoeopathic Arnica and Symphytum on his lips. Next thing I knew the head nurse was striding across the room pointing at me with a doctor in tow. The doctor was polite and wanted to know what I was putting in his mouth. I explained that I was a very experienced herbalist that I was merely giving Tom a few drops of a homoeopathic remedy for shock and that I had the support of the father and mother for what I was doing. He said, 'We are in charge here and we are responsible for him, not the father and mother. No one is allowed to do anything without our permission'.

I looked into the eyes of this specialist and said, 'We are both working to save the life of this boy. Not just the life but the quality of his life. I promise you that I know what I am doing and I am contributing to your work. You have saved his life. My work will help him recover faster and end up in better condition. I am very experienced. I can provide details of my membership of two professional associations. I can give you the phone numbers of clients who have been with me for years. I teach herbal medicine at tertiary institutes. Please let me help to save this boy'.

He said, 'I need to be sure you are not using anything blood thinning—like Arnica. And don't put anything else in his mouth. It's not just my decision. There are a team of specialists who must be consulted. Now you have to stop treating him'.

I pleaded, 'Can you call a meeting of them? I will talk to them. Please give me a chance to use my medicine to help this boy. Look at him. He needs everything we can all do'. I kept looking him in the eyes. Tears were rolling down my cheeks. 'Okay', he said. 'At 11 am tomorrow I will call them all together and you can discuss it with them. Please make sure the parents are with you'.

I hardly slept that night. I made phone calls to friends who were osteopaths and herbalists to ask for their advice and maybe to get them to email me scientific studies about herbs I had in my mixes for Tom. Planning what to say that night I realised that nothing would help my case in the morning. To try and explain to them that the actions of homoeopathic Arnica cannot be described as blood thinning—would be a waste of time.

My understanding of their medicine is that each drug has one main action—which switches something off or stimulates one process or mimics something in the body. Simple but very powerful medicine. The repercussions and side effects of each drug used are very strong. Where was the basis for a conversation in which we could understand each other? Their medicine can keep this almost-dead body alive while my medicine repairs gently with natural ingredients that have no life-threatening side effects. Quietly in the night I understood some of the reasons they are afraid of my medicine.

If I told them how many actions each herb has, they might panic and consider it to be threateningly uncontrollable. They think we have no idea what we are doing and what doses we should use. I think that they have very little idea of how to repair a human body or how to work out doses appropriate for the individual. My work is regularly to help repair bodies that are suffering the side effects of modern drugs and their work is emergency work which can save lives.

Their work is so dangerous that their insurance is massive. What a lot of pressure they have. Of course, they are afraid of someone coming in and treating the body alongside them. They have all the power and all the responsibility. Unless power of attorney has been sorted out to take the responsibility back where it should belong—to the patient and the person closest to them—responsibility goes with power, power over ourselves and our own lives.

The dreaded meeting time came. Marina and John were still deep in shock. Five male specialists and nervous me. I waited for them to start. They all looked at each other and finally appointed one amongst them to begin. He did.

'Well, we've decided that we don't mind you using all these oils. They are obviously making you feel that you are helping him. The smell is annoying some of the nursing staff but that's just the strong Lavender. We think they are harmless but we won't allow you to put anything into his mouth'. As I sighed with relief, Marina said, 'We want you to know that we want her help and so would Tom if he could speak'. All I said was, 'Thank you'.

They waited a few seconds for us to speak more, looked a bit surprised, looked at each other, 'Well, if that's all then we should get back to work'. Hurriedly I spoke again. 'Thank you. We are very grateful that you have taken the time to meet with us and allow us to continue helping in this way. Thank you'.

That night the head nurse was annoyed that we were still using the oils. She tried to stop us. Over the top of Tom's body she told us she didn't like the smell and we were to stop immediately. I told her we had permission and support from the specialists. I stared her down and kept applying the oils with herbs in. The nurse ended up shouting at me. 'How dare you look at me like that. I'll make sure you get stopped!' Then she strode off. Marina and I both shook with distress.

Mid-afternoon on the third day we were invited to a meeting about Tom's treatment. Marina and John asked me to stay with them and we met with three specialists. They told us Tom's progress was so good that they thought he was able to cope with an operation to install plates all over his head to reconnect his face, nose, and jaw to the back of his skull. It sounded very complex. I could see that Marina and John in their shocked state had no idea how to have this discussion.

I asked, 'How many plates do you need to install on Tom's skull and where? What exactly will you have to do to Tom to install them?' They told us in detail. I watched Marina and John start to shake and I realised I had to be careful with my questions. 'How long will the anaesthetic need to last for such a complex operation?'

'Four or five hours', one of them replied.

I was worried. 'Don't you think that this is too close to the accident for such a long anaesthetic and such a very complex operation? Don't you think his body is in such deep shock that this is dangerous? Can't we wait another week for this operation?'

'Yes, it is a bit close to the accident but the best surgeon for this job is available today and may not be so available in a few days. We think that Tom is doing well enough to handle it. We weren't expecting such good progress, but now we think he is young enough and strong enough to cope'.

At the same time as John spoke, I said, 'Can we take an hour in private to make this decision?' And John said, 'We agree to him having this operation today. We accept your advice and we want you to do what you think is best'.

Marina knew I was worried. We went for a walk and I told her why in the most basic way I could.

> *A shock such as Tom's accident completely empties the adrenal glands of the body where all the vital force of the human being is stored. It leaves the body locked in the state of terror the body has achieved seconds before loss of consciousness comes. Our adrenal glands, with the hormones they produce, control our most vital functions, such as heartbeat, blood pressure, circulation, metabolism of blood sugar for energy, blood supply to muscles, pain relief and anti-inflammatory activity.*
>
> *An anaesthetic empties the adrenal glands to put the body into the kind of unconsciousness that closes down all the vital functions. It is like the very edge of death. Recovering from this is similar to recovering from*

> severe shock. Tom has had a terrible accident, a massive operation the following day, and now looks like having another one three days after the accident. I believe this operation will take longer than four or five hours and that he may not be able to survive it. It would be better for Tom if we had longer to get him ready for this operation.

Marina didn't seem to have the strength to deal with this and I realised that I had given her more to worry about when we still didn't know if Tom was going to ever come out of his coma or be a normal person again. I went in to see Tom with a heavy heart but I treated him with oils, herbs, flower essences, and homoeopathy, and I talked to him about the operation and how to handle it. I gave him Reiki and told him that all my treatments would have made him strong enough to get through it. I told him he could do it and that we would all be there with him during the operation and ready to resume treating him afterwards. Then I went home to the Blue Mountains to my herb garden and cried for hours and then slept.

I left all my treatments with Marina with lots of instructions. I was exhausted and crazy with worry. I needed to get my negative energy out of their vicinity and clean it up before I could go back. I knew too much and the responsibility of this knowledge was too much for me. I knew that my presence in the hospital that day had become extra stress for them. How could I go on in this friendship if I hadn't given everything I could to the recovery of this precious boy?

While I slept in my own bed Tom came to visit me. In my dreams he cried and begged me to come back. He told me he needed me to help him heal. Just like when he was the challenging, cheeky 2-year-old, he wanted to stand behind me and be protected. In my dream I cried and said I didn't know if I was strong enough. He said he couldn't do it without me. I woke up crying.

The phone rang. It was Marina sobbing. She said the operation had been nine hours and they'd nearly lost him on the operating table. She said he looked terrible again. His head was three times normal size again and his body felt empty. I told her she had to start immediately using all my treatments. She said, 'I can't. I'm afraid to. I'm afraid that I'll cause more trouble with the nurses'.

I was worried. 'This is your son. You have the right to help him in any way that you can. Do you want him to die? I'll be back in three hours'.

I made myself some mixes to strengthen myself and drove back the long drive to Kogarah. I resolved to try and keep my own anxiety contained. Tom needed me and only I knew just how much could be done with my mixes. No point talking about it or thinking someone else could do it. I arrived at the hospital and resumed my treatment of Tom. It was the fourth day. He responded beautifully.

That afternoon they said he was doing so well that the next morning they would try and bring him out of coma. 'We need to reduce the medication which is keeping him sedated and find out if he can come out of his coma. If he can be brought out he will think that he is at the scene of the accident and he could be very upset and possibly angry'. They said we couldn't be present because it might be too distressing to watch.

Tom was able to come out of the coma but was so distressed they sedated him again. Over the next two days he was brought out of coma many times. Each time got easier and then we were allowed to be present for one of the times. He recognised us and it helped him. The terror in his eyes took many days to calm down. He was quickly able to communicate yes and no.

They came and warned us not to be hopeful. 'You must understand that the brain damage from the accident was so severe that it could be many months before we know if he will ever be normal. When he can move around better we will move him to a brain rehabilitation unit where he will embark on brain physiotherapy treatment. This can take a long time, anything up to a year. He may never remember the accident and he may have trouble remembering his friends and even yourselves. How much of his memory will come back we don't know. He will have to relearn even how to control his body'.

We were sure he knew us. We asked him and he responded. He tried many times to pull the tubes out of his nose, mouth, throat, and lungs. Tom the rebel was back! We encouraged the nurses to finally have them removed on day seven. At last, we could expect him to talk. And he did. Each time he woke up we were there. Marina, with love and patience, talked him through these steps every time: 'Where are you? Who are you? Do you know why you are here? Do you know who I am? Do you know what is wrong with your body?'

At first, she had to give him the answers. Within hours he was giving the answers with his own jokes added on. Her questions got more complicated. When she asked him who I was he replied, 'Well, it's not Buddy. It must be Linda'. Buddy was his dog—who hadn't been mentioned at the hospital. We had some memory back!

Once he could speak and demonstrate he knew what was going on (the eighth day after the accident), we could ask him if he wanted herbal medicines to take by mouth. I had them ready. He pointed to me. 'If they're yours I want them'. I gave them to him—mixes designed to clear deep bruising, mend broken bones, repair circulation, clear fluid leaked out and trapped in tissue, repair adrenal function, and restore everything. They were the same herbs I had in the oil mixes we had applied, which sent them in through the circulation. Now we could send them in through his digestive system as well. If held under the tongue they would go straight to the brain.

His right arm had been causing him a lot of pain and his neck brace was very uncomfortable. His ability to respond to conversation was hampered by high doses of morphine. So on the ninth day I asked him if he wanted to try herbal medicines for the pain. He did. They worked for him without the side effects of morphine—which had been fogging his brain and causing him to lapse into dulled sleepiness and depression. With the first dose of herbs, he said to me, 'Aaaargh, the taste of those herbs hasn't got any better'. We laughed. Then he grabbed my arm and looked me in the eyes. 'Thanks for coming back', he said.

On the 12th day, he was sitting in a comfy chair and making jokes but restless and uncomfortable with the neck brace, trying to pull it off. Marina told him he wasn't to remove it. I suggested she go and have a coffee with Alice while I gave Tom some Reiki. She went. Tom looked me in the eyes and reached up to pull at his neck brace. I knew from past experience that the herbs I'd given him to repair bone could do it in two weeks—without a trace of the break on an X-ray. I'd seen it a number of times with clients. So I said, 'Tom, there is a strong chance that your neck is closer to being healed than anyone realises so … if I tip the chair back so you are lying down and you promise to keep your head, neck, and shoulders still, I'll let you take the neck brace off for five minutes'.

I was giving him Reiki when Marina arrived back. She stood in the doorway and told us both, 'You shouldn't have that neck brace off. The doctors will be very upset and you shouldn't have let him take it off'. Under my hands, I could feel Tom's strong energy. One of the doctors appeared behind Marina. 'That's a very stupid thing to do, young man. You'll need to wear that brace for at least six months or you'll risk more injury'. As he spoke, under my hands I could feel Tom's energy shrinking into hopelessness.

The doctor left. Marina and Alice announced it was lunchtime. Tom was wiped out. I asked Tom if he wanted lunch, or Reiki and me talking to his body while he dozed. He said he wanted me to work on him. Marina and Alice went to get lunch. Under my hands, Tom quickly dropped into a light sleep as I talked. I told him it was up to him how quickly he got better. No one else could predict this. I told him stories of how fast the herbs had helped my clients. I told him how strong he was and what a miracle it was for him to be this much recovered already and I told him that awful neck brace would be gone soon. While I was talking to his subconscious with my hands on his injured body, or just giving Reiki, I could feel powerful energies flowing back into his body.

After three and a half weeks in the St George Emergency Care Unit, no one could find any reason to keep him there or to send him for brain rehabilitation. They sent him home to Coffs Harbour Hospital to be near home until he was well enough to go home. He still had a neck brace on and a plastered left leg. After two weeks there they couldn't find any reason to keep the neck brace on, or the leg plaster. They took them off and sent him home. He spent Christmas running around the countryside happy to be alive, wild again and sober, loving his friends and showing them his scars. No more drinking and no more motorbikes for him. The fear will stay for a long time.

He told me in a quiet conversation that he remembered some of the things I said to him while he was in that coma. He told me things I'd said that no one else heard. He remembered being out in space with the spiritual healers too—he described it. And he knew he'd visited me in my dream. He told me what he'd said.

I loved working alongside those dedicated doctors and nursing staff. I know they kept his body alive. I know how fantastic their system is in such an emergency. And I know Tom would still be very damaged without my medicine. This opportunity that I was given to be protected and trusted as a member of the family while I helped to repair someone I love was a great privilege.

For Tom I had prepared a mix of the flower essences: Rescue Remedy (Bach Flower Remedy) mixed with Vital Spark, Healing, Renaissance (Himalayan Flower Enhancers) and Wendy Forbes' Humanifest flower and gem essences, all in one bottle. I had also added some homoeopathic liquids: Arnica, Symphytum, and Hypericum. As well, I had prepared a mix to apply to his injuries with specific herbal tinctures (including Comfrey) added to infused Hypericum oil plus small amounts of Lavender and Rosemary essential oils. To this I'd added small amounts of Vital Spark, other Himalayan Flower Enhancers, and homoeopathic Arnica, Symphytum, and Hypericum.

St George Hospital Emergency Care Unit was a sad, all-white sort of place. Like the set of a science fiction movie. A sea of cold, silent beds filled with cold, silent bodies in deep comas on life support machines. No music, no laughter, no loving visitors, no prayers. No whispering in ears. No herbs, no oils, no Rescue Remedy, and no herbalists. No life anywhere. [More details about the herbs and dosages used in this story are detailed in Chapter 24, page 137.]

CHAPTER FIVE

A vicious assault—Andrew's story

Andrew is Rose's son. He is 6 foot 6 inches tall—one of those gentle giants we talk about. One Friday night Andy was having a drink with his mates in the pub after work. While he was happily chatting away to his friends, little did he know that a psychotic man was heading his way, visiting almost every town in the Blue Mountains and assaulting people as he went.

When this man got to the pub Andy was in, he grabbed a billiard cue and swung it at the back of Andy's head. It connected hard across the base of his skull. He went down like a tonne of bricks and hit the back of his head on the billiard table edge on the way.

The ambulance came and Andy was fighting for his life. His brain was bleeding into his lungs. He stayed in a coma for five days. Rose, his mother, rang me from the hospital on the first morning and told me about it. 'We need some herbs, kid. What can you give us? I know you can help. This is my son and they don't know if he will survive or ever be normal again. I'm coming home briefly this afternoon—can I collect something to help?' I had no idea if I could help but I knew I had to try.

Rose arrived. She cried a lot. I gave her Rescue Remedy and hot, sweet tea. Andy's wife was still at the hospital and Andy was in the ICU—with rigorous supervision. I'd prepared a mix of herbs that

I thought would help, and a bottle of Rescue Remedy. I told her to put the Rescue Remedy in his mouth and to rub it on his temples and head every hour as close to the injury as possible.

His wife wouldn't let Rose put anything in his mouth, even 10 drops of Rescue Remedy. So when Andy's wife was out of the room Rose used the Rescue Remedy. She was too worried about the wife's reactions to use the herbs. They needed bigger doses and this might cause him to choke. Also, she didn't want to cause problems with the staff if she was discovered.

Andy came out of his coma after five days, and two and a half weeks later he came out of hospital. He still hadn't had any herbs but he was conscious and lucid and asked for me to visit him at home. I went. His wife was there to help him give me the details I needed. His speech was a bit of a struggle.

It was Thursday. He'd stopped most of his tablets on Tuesday when he came out of hospital. He'd been on a lot, including antibiotics just in case he got an infection. 'Where they put the canula in my arm it got infected all the way up to the elbow. It was very painful. And I had a partial seizure while in hospital so they put me on lots of codeine products and I haven't been able to sleep since. Without them, I've got a bad headache so I've been taking Panadol for two days and have been able to sleep better and the headache is only low level now. I'm badly constipated, haven't been for four days. Better give me some herbs for that as well!'

Andy still had blood and fluid on the brain—and brain swelling. 'I'm still on the pills for that but I want to get off them. I want you to do it with herbs. Can you do it? They told me they thought my brain might not be able to clear any more out. That the clearing was done in the first week or so and I might be stuck with what's left in there'.

The assault had caused two blood vessels to burst and bleed into the front of his head behind the forehead, and from the back of the head the damage had caused the leak into the lungs. The swelling was affecting his short-term memory, but not his long-term memory. He was slow talking and shaky but easy to understand. 'And I've got like a buzzing in my ears which changes as I move my head around, sounds like a mozzie. It's pretty boring'.

I mixed up some herbal tinctures with oil, Hypericum infused in almond oil. I didn't add Rescue Remedy because I knew he'd had lots of it already. My intention was that the oils would carry the tinctures in through the skin and start to clean up the fluids and blood in the brain that shouldn't be there. I thought of it like treating bad bruises.

I also made a herbal mix for him to take by mouth, to repair him from the inside. I told him to take 4 ml four times daily. He decided to stop taking the doctor's pills. He didn't tell me for two weeks. I had encouraged him not to stop them. I told him my medicine would work regardless and it was better to have the backup of the pharmaceuticals.

Two weeks later Andy went for an ultrasound—no more fluid or blood was stuck in the brain. He was feeling much better—no headaches, no mozzie-like tinnitus, improved speaking ability, improved body control, and no constipation. 'If I miss a dose I start getting a headache and I take it five times daily. I feel real good on it'. I made him repeat mixes, checking each time for any other difficult symptoms that may need help from the herb mix.

Two and half months later he let himself run out of herbs to see how he felt. He rang me. 'I didn't get any headaches but the tinnitus is creeping back in and I've been a bit depressed. The doc suggested some antidepressants and I told him I'd rather take your herbs. So I wanna stay on them for a while longer'.

Andy was on my herbal mixes for a year. He was back at work eight weeks after the assault.

CHAPTER SIX

Herbs and hearts — Ruby's story

Early in my career as a qualified herbalist (in 1985), I drove from Balmain, in Sydney, to Kurrajong mountain each week to give a talk to the guests of the Kurrajong Health Retreat. After my talk, I was available to consult with whoever made an appointment that day.

One day a young woman of 17 arrived at my door. Pale and frail, with no energy field at all, she sat outside humbly and waited. I'll never forget her. She had undergone open heart surgery 18 months before, at age 15, and couldn't quite remember why. Since leaving hospital she had been afraid to go out of the house and felt like she had no interest in anything. She found it hard to get up in the morning, and only did so because it upset her mother if she didn't.

After months of this listlessness, her doctor had put her on an antidepressant. Since then she had no interest in eating and felt nauseous all the time. She lived in Sydney with her mother. Her father had left them a year before her open heart surgery. I did my best to convince her to come and see me for a follow-up back in Sydney but I never saw her again.

During the drive back down into Sydney I remembered how I felt after my dad left us when I was 13. And I wondered how I would feel after being thrown around an operating theatre, slashed open down the middle and peeled back like a spatchcock while a team of people readjusted what they thought was wrong with my heart. Of course, you are unconscious. Well, you are anaesthetised.

Actually, you are in a state of hovering on the brink of death—this is what the anaesthetic does, switches off your vital force; your blood pressure, heart rate, metabolism, and energy production are all brought to an almost standstill. However, since your awareness exists in all your cells and in the unconscious of your brain, you are aware of what is happening to you and you are helpless. The terror is held in your unconscious and then allowed expression upon consciousness revival. That's why people can cry for days after an anaesthetic, or go into terror on waking up from a coma following an accident.

About 12 years later, in October 1995, a woman brought her 18-year-old daughter to me with a very serious problem. She felt like she'd tried everything. She was a skilled naturopath herself and had researched her daughter's problem and had her daughter on a range of supplements.

We'll call her daughter Ruby. The problem, the episodes, had been getting worse for four years. The diagnosis of it by a heart specialist was 'superventrical tachycardia' and 'ectopic arrhythmia'. The episodes were becoming extreme attacks, and were increasing—she'd had four in five months—and during the attacks she actually died in the ambulance on the way to hospital.

The heart specialist had figured out that Ruby had two electrical pulses in the heart instead of one. These pulses control the heartbeat. This specialist advised mother and daughter that open heart surgery was needed to cut out one of the electrical controls and after this there would be no more tachycardia and no more emergencies. He considered that her attacks were part of the double heartbeat pumping too much blood into her heart and that this blood spilt over into her lungs, preventing her from breathing—and so she died, drowning in her own blood, during the attacks, and needed major emergency resuscitation.

I asked Ruby when the arrhythmias started. This is what she told me: 'I've had heart arrhythmias for a long time. They started four years ago when I had viral hepatitis and an Epstein-Barr virus (shingles) at the same time. I was off school for a few months. Then six months after I started to feel better I got a bad dose of chickenpox. So I went into chronic fatigue syndrome and mum had me on a lot of supplements. I had to give up school and I think without the supplements I wouldn't be able to work. I've got a part-time job that I love in a health shop. I get

HERBS AND HEARTS — RUBY'S STORY   45

sick a lot with bronchitis and tummy flu. I feel nauseous a lot of the time. At one stage mum gave me kombucha drinks and the arrhythmia increased so I stopped taking them'.

I asked Ruby to describe the symptoms leading to the attacks. She said, 'Early on, before they became so serious, I just had regular breathing difficulties. Like I forgot to breathe. And I'd get a fullness in my chest with a burning feeling in the centre, just above my breasts, like there's something in the way of me breathing. No dizziness. If I sat down and relaxed I would be able to breathe again slowly'.

This sounded like a kind of asthma to me—adrenal stress and deficiency of magnesium—which leads to inability of muscles to contract or relax. I asked her if she got muscle cramps or twitches anywhere in her body. 'Yes I do. I have aching legs all the time and regular painful muscle spasms and cramps in my calves. And I have broken blood vessels already in my legs. I get muscle twitches all the time here in the surface skin around my heart'.

Her mother described her as extremely sensitive and emotionally vulnerable. Ruby claimed to be anxious a lot, said she got itchy arms and lumpy elbows which she thought was stress-related—part of her constant feeling of anxiety. I'd be anxious too if my heart was doing what hers was. Or *was* it her heart?

I asked her to describe the severe attacks and where they started. 'They start here, just above my waist at the front. It's like a flush, warm and getting hotter, like a wave. The arrhythmia/tachycardia is part of it and that gets more intense. Then I get the other symptoms as well, the breathing difficulties, and I get very dizzy. I have to lie down or I'll fall down. Now when I lie down I hope someone is calling an ambulance because soon after that I pass out'.

I asked Ruby how long she thought she had between the beginning of the attack and passing out? She thought she had between ten to 20 minutes. I asked her if there was an increase in feeling nauseous before the symptoms started. Yes, there was.

I went into my dispensary and prayed for help. More than anything else I wanted to help that young woman avoid heart surgery. I didn't believe it would help. I made a mix of herbs to support her immune system to recover from the chronic fatigue—it had liver herbs to repair the viral damage as well as antiviral herbs. I put her on 1 ml four times daily. She was taking magnesium and Echinacea. I increased her magnesium.

Then I made a mix designed to treat all the symptoms of the heart, lung, adrenal glands, stomach, and muscle difficulties she'd described to me as her 'attacks'. I put her on 30 drops four times daily. I explained that it was designed to repair all aspects of these crises and that as soon as she felt any increase in nausea or difficulty breathing or the beginning of the flushing she was to take a whole dropper full (approximately 30 drops) of the mix and 10 drops every five minutes until she was sure she was going to be okay. I asked her to phone me straightaway if she had to use the emergency dosing, and then we would review the treatment and dosing.

I didn't hear from Ruby for three weeks. I phoned her. She was doing fine with no threats of her 'attacks'. She came back when her herbs were nearly finished—two months later.

She told me, 'I haven't once forgotten to breathe. The chest fullness and burning has gone and I haven't felt there is something in the way of breathing at all. I haven't been nauseous, not once. I haven't had heart arrhythmias at all while standing up and only once have I had them lying down. It happened a couple of weeks ago when I got into bed after two full and busy days at work in the shop. I took some extra herbs and was fine in minutes. And last night in the car I got lost and panicked a bit, then I got a little wave of the flushing with a bit of a red neck and face. It wasn't intense and went away before I had a chance to stop the car and get my herbs out'.

Ruby and I worked on her recovery from the severe viral infections for three years. Along with her other herbs she continued to take 'Heart Mix 1' for all this time. As long as she had this mix with her in her handbag, she felt strong and sure of survival. She didn't have anything wrong with her heart after all. I wonder what the heart surgeon would have done with Ruby opened up on the table and no second electrical pulse to cut out? What would he have told Ruby and her mum afterwards? And would she have survived this dramatic surgery?

After two years of building up her strength with herbal mixes and supplements, Ruby took over as manager of the health shop. Then after another two years of working and saving, she went on an overseas trip. She didn't need to take Heart Mix 1 with her. Every one to two years Ruby, or her mum, contact me to let me know she is still fine—almost 30 years later. She has a family of her own and I can see her on Facebook, happy and healthy and living a full life. [More details about the herbs and dosages used in this story are detailed in Chapter 24, page 137.]

CHAPTER SEVEN

Can you save my leg?—Klaus's story

*T**he following story is straight from the pen of a young Norwegian who became my friend after I treated him—Klaus Roberg, Physiotherapist and Chiropractor. This is what he experienced, in his own words.*

The closest I have ever been to an amputation happened in 2006. I was 28 years old and studying chiropractic in Sydney, a long way from Norway where I grew up. One weekend in April I went on a trip to explore the great Australian Outback with three other Norwegians, one Italian, and an Aussie friend called Simon. He had been talking a lot about how vast everything was out there, and how much fun we could have, so when his uncle went away on vacation, he invited us to stay at his uncle's farm for the weekend. We drove past the Blue Mountains and into unknown territory for the Norwegian–Italian squad.

After driving on a road that stretched out for ages, we finally got to this little town in the middle of nowhere, where the local pub had nothing but trophy fish on all the walls. We Norwegians are used to isolated places, but the Outback gave the concept a whole new dimension.

On the last day of the trip, we got to ride his uncle's old dirt bikes around on the big farm. I was the only one who actually owned a motorbike at that time, so I got the oldest one. It didn't respond quite as it should, and after a while I got thrown off and I managed to get a long and deep cut on my left front shin. I knew it wasn't good news when I could see the bone of my tibia as I lay on the ground.

The small local hospital didn't want to stitch me up before I had taken an X-ray at a bigger hospital, but they offered me as much morphine as I wanted, which I politely declined as I wasn't in that much pain. It turned out the bone wasn't affected, so they stitched me up and sent me back to Sydney with some antibiotics.

After ten days, I went to a GP as instructed, and he wasn't very impressed when he opened the dressing and found an infection in the wound. It had a rather smelly odour, and quite a bit of pus. He took a blood sample and gave me another antibiotic. As a chiropractic student, I was aware of the risk of bone infection, and when I went back after another week and it looked even worse; I started to get seriously worried.

The third antibiotic didn't do any good either, and I had no clue what to do in order to reverse the process or at least slow it down. At that time I was attending a few seminars and I remember practising one of the techniques when the teacher came over and noticed the covered-up wound. He almost got sick when he had a look and could smell the odour from it.

The following weekend I did an Applied Kinesiology seminar with a gentleman called Keith Keen. He had recently had open heart surgery, and was going on about how well the scars were healing, all thanks to this woman called Linda Bates who had given him some ointments for the wound to heal faster and better.

I knew I had to get her number, and called her the day afterwards. I was still a bit sceptical, but I was hoping she at least could give me something to slow down the infection so the antibiotics could work better. Thankfully, I got an appointment the day after I called her, and I remember thinking about what would happen to me if she couldn't help, and neither could any doctor. I realised I could be close to having my leg amputated just below the knee. I love to go running in the mountains and do all sorts of sports and activities, and the thought of not being able to continue with all my passions was not pleasant at all.

Linda looked quite concerned after getting the whole story and when she had a look at the sick-looking wound. But she said she was quite certain that she could help me, and she made several ointments and herb mixes for me to apply to the wound and a large tincture mix for me to drink several times per day. It didn't taste particularly good as I recall, but not all healthy things do taste good. I was supposed to change the bandages two times per day to apply more herbs each time and take regular baths in the ocean because of the good properties of salt.

On the third day, I started noticing the first small changes. The wound looked slightly less red and a little bit less swollen. That was when I realised that the stuff was actually working! I got more and more excited every day, and by the fifth day I could see how the wound was healing hour by hour.

By the end of the first week, there was no pus left, and the wound was closing. After ten days of this treatment, the wound finally closed itself. I never went back to the GP who had prescribed three antibiotic treatments so far with no result. But I did go back to Linda Bates for a few follow-ups.

During my first year in Australia, I had managed to get some problems with my digestion, and had severe stomach pain because of that, partly because I was stressed for long periods due to all the exams I had to pass. Linda gave me herbal medicine for that as well, and shortly after I finally felt I had good levels of energy for the first time in years.

The leg injury healed gradually over the next two months until the scar was as good as any other scar. I know for sure that there would have been a serious high chance of complications if Linda hadn't done her magic, and I am truly grateful for all she has done for me. The story didn't end with just me being as good as new again because it turned out Linda is only one week older than my mother, and I felt like she was my second mum when I was so far away from my family in Norway.

So we kept in touch and I was very happy when she finally decided to come and visit Norway and my family in July 2012. I remember her genuine excitement at seeing medicinal plants growing all over the city of Bergen, and lots in my garden. She spent several weeks consulting patients at my clinic, and her vast knowledge of herbal medicine is something I greatly miss over here.

CHAPTER EIGHT

No more surgery needed—Anita's story

It was January 2004, eight months after Anita's second hip replacement operation. At dinner I watched Anita struggle to eat. Both her hands were swollen at the wrists and finger joints. The middle joints of the fingers were bent at right angles. 'I have to wear splints at night to try and straighten them', she said. Her head and neck appeared fixed, head tilted to one side. To look around she had to turn her whole upper body. Walking was stiff and clumsy, her torso swaying to help her lift each leg in turn. Psoriatic arthritis, her mother had told me.

I'd first met Anita at her mother's house in 1999. She was 24 then. A tall, graceful young woman, making her way in the world with confidence. After travelling and working in England and Europe during 1996 and 1997 she returned to Australia, and by 2002 she had completed a teaching degree. I didn't see her in the intervening years but her mother had told me about the sudden onset and progression of this illness, in 2002, and some of Anita's history. While Anita was having hip replacement surgery, in mid-2003, her mother regularly confided concern for her daughter's future.

That morning, after I watched Anita awkwardly trying to eat, I heard her bumping around gathering her things to depart for her home. Her partner was taking luggage to the car while Anita was dispensing her daily medications—Prednisone, Methotrexate, Celebrex, and the oral contraceptive pill.

I went to the door of the room. 'Please forgive me if I'm intruding but I can't listen to you dispensing all these tablets without asking if you'd like my help with your recovery? Please tell me if I'm out of line'. Anita sighed. 'You're my mother's close friend and I didn't want to impose but I'd love your help'.

Back at the dining table, we talked for half an hour. I gave her my travelling container of a supplement powder I'd been travelling with (designed for anti-inflammatory action). 'Take 1 teaspoon three times daily. We'll talk on the phone in two days when we're both home'.

I thought about Anita all the way to my home in the Blue Mountains. What did I know about her history? I only knew what her mother had told me. She was the eldest child and when she was 3 years old her mother gave birth to a boy. Anita loved him and very soon was sleeping in the bed with him. Before his first birthday, this little boy was diagnosed with cancer and the family began that distressing time filled with worry, prayers, chemotherapy, and endless visits to specialists.

Anita still insisted on sleeping with him and this seemed to comfort them both. Just before his third birthday, he died in his father's arms while Anita was at school. She was six years old and heartbroken. Within three months of his death, she'd managed to become a brave little girl; she also had the beginnings of psoriasis and difficulty eating certain foods. The house was filled with grief and she couldn't help, no matter how hard she tried.

The psoriasis continued on her belly, elbows, backs of her knees, and sometimes on her upper arms. It wasn't a big problem then. The patches were small and sometimes it healed completely—but not for long. Her mother and father had a veggie garden and were using fresh, organic whole foods. When she was 8 years old her mother gave birth to another boy. This made her happy.

Her parents separated when she was 12 years old. Three months later she fell ill with scarlet fever—a strain of streptococcal (bacterial) infection. *Pears Encyclopaedia of Child Health* says 'Scarlet fever is focused in the lymph nodes around the throat and neck, armpits, sides of chest and groin. Sometimes it involves lymph around the bowel, inside the lower abdomen. Rare complications lead to rheumatic fever'.

Anita's scarlet fever became rheumatic fever and she was severely ill for four months. Her mother reports her being unable to walk for most of this time; she had to crawl to the bathroom. The only allopathic treatment was antibiotics, for months. During this time her psoriasis became severe, covering her lower abdomen, upper arms, thighs, and upper chest, and her digestive difficulties increased.

As Anita recovered from scarlet fever, she contracted a bad dose of chickenpox—one of the Epstein-Barr family of viruses—a virus which thrives in the nervous system and skin, producing painful sores. Chickenpox came again when Anita was 15. Both episodes took her four to six weeks in bed to recover. Allopathic medicine had no treatment for chicken pox, only anti-inflammatory painkillers.

The day after I arrived back home to the Blue Mountains I rang Anita. She reported good results from taking the powder I had given her—less pain, and the inflammation in her joints had gone down a little. This told me that we had a good chance of working together with herbs and supplements to repair her body. I knew it would take a lot of regular time and energy from me for a long time. This young woman was yet again too sick to be able to work. How would I help her feel okay about this? How would I get her involved in her own healing?

I thought deeply about this. The next day I rang her again. I told her I would do the work with her for no charge with the following conditions: 'I want you to keep a journal of your progress and maybe we can make a book together about your healing. I want you to phone me every week till we know we have made breakthroughs and then I want you to phone me every time you feel like you are going backwards. I want you to journal your dreams, collect the doctor's test results, keep meditating, make notes on how your body responds to diet, supplements and herb mixes, and dedicate yourself to doing what we agree you need to do. This will teach us both heaps and I will enjoy sharing your healing journey. Think about it and I'll call you back tomorrow'.

Anita replied, 'I don't have to think about it. I'd love your help and will be happy to do what you ask. I have already been writing a journal over the last three years—it's my way of releasing my body from the emotional stress I hold. Thank you'. I said, 'Okay, great. So let's make a time to start—we need about two to three hours on the phone first off. I need your history so gather your notes'. We made a time for our first detailed talk.

I phoned Anita's mother to make sure this was all okay with her. She was thrilled. I told her my main concern. 'This is going to cost a lot in herbal medicines and supplements and it could take a few years. How do you think Anita will manage this?' She replied, 'I don't want her to have to worry about this, or you either. I will arrange this and I'd like to make sure none of this creates anything that will damage our friendship. If anything begins to be difficult, will you please let me know?' I promised I would.

At first, it was very hard to get a breakthrough. We began with diet. I had to help her remove all possible causes of inflammation from her daily consumption. I knew from her increase in psoriasis during the scarlet fever that Anita was most likely allergic to the sulphur used in many antibiotics. Her response to sulphur was inflammation. She had to study the ingredients list on every product and change her shopping habits to eliminate food additives, preservatives (many of them are sulphates), colourings, and flavourings.

She did this with enthusiasm and cleaned out the pantry, 'I know it helps because I went to a naturopath in England for 12 months and my health improved lots. She asked me to avoid all food additives and eat fresh whole foods too'.

I also asked her to carefully follow her blood type diet—concentrating on eating mostly foods that are highly beneficial. This meant no wheat or dairy and some of her special favourites—like potatoes. It took three to four months for Anita to directly experience and clearly realise what happened to her when she couldn't resist things like just a few Jatz crackers [containing wheat] with cheese at informal get-togethers. The joint swelling and pain took two or three days to become obvious and then remained for one to two weeks. Slowly, through pain, Anita lost all interest in these foods.

While giving me her history she talked about her years at college. She was 17 and living away from home. Sometimes processed wheat and sugary foods were all she ate for days. She had regular digestive pain and psoriasis then. As she finished her teaching qualification Anita came down with glandular fever, followed by arthritis in her right hand. The following winter her psoriasis and arthritis flared badly. Homoeopathic treatment helped calm it down.

At that first consultation in mid-February, it was hard to work out what was going on in Anita's body. I looked up the drugs and read about the side effects. I needed to try and work out the symptoms and the causes of her psoriasis and joint inflammation before I could begin treatment because the drugs would be covering up the symptoms I wanted to hear about. Also, I needed to work out which herbs would have the anti-inflammatory pain relief effect which would stop the disintegration of bones and tendons in Anita's joints. The medications she was taking didn't seem to be reducing swelling or inflammation but they covered up the pain. And they gave her side effects—a whole new range of symptoms.

Anita was so afraid of the pain that she took more Celebrex or Panadol to stop it. I needed to hear about the pain—what time of day was it the worst?; did it get worse after eating?; how many hours after eating?; what did it feel like first thing in the morning?; did heat help or make it worse?; did it feel hot inside the joints?

As long as she stayed on painkillers I could not get answers to these and many other questions. Did she get headaches? *She wouldn't feel them.* Did she have digestive pain and inflammation? *She wouldn't feel it.* How did she sleep? *She could be simply knocked out on medications that stopped nerve signals.*

Depressed, overwhelmed, trapped, and very worried about how she would cope in the future: this was how Anita felt. Since she seemed to be in so much pain, even with the medications, was she to be forever at the mercy of modern medicine and dependent on her specialists? She had new hips and still could hardly move without pain and effort. She felt disempowered and regularly felt she didn't want to live like this.

In mid-February 2004 Anita started taking herbal medicines and naturopathic supplements for anti-inflammatory pain relief and repair. She put the oral contraceptive pill in the bin and dedicated herself to her own recovery. She chose not to discuss any of it with her specialists for fear that they would abandon her.

According to her blood test results the inflammatory markers were not changing much with her drug regime and her specialists had predicted she would need knee replacements by mid-2005. She felt that the pharmaceutical drugs were damaging her and she wanted to work towards coming off them.

For Anita, a regular meditation practice was very beneficial. An hour daily helped her release emotional tension and the tightness that was contributing to pain inside and around the swollen joints. Taking up a part-time teaching job to help satisfy her need to work and contribute to society, Anita found that in school holidays, once or twice a year, she would attend a meditation retreat and this helped her make important breakthroughs in letting go of emotional baggage that she felt had been contributing to her illness.

In these early days, regular exercise wasn't possible. I suggested acupuncture for its ability to heal and reconnect the nervous system and this too helped. I also recommended treatment with a particular Doctor of Chiropractic who uses Applied Kinesiology to investigate the causes of problems—emotional, biochemical deficiencies, metabolic pathways, and heavy metal toxicity.

This method can be very precise in working out treatments and testing the body for solutions of a biochemical, homoeopathic, naturopathic, or herbal nature. One treatment every three or four months helped Anita unravel more layers of causes and to release tensions in muscle groups that were keeping her body in painful stress. From the first treatment she reported more movement in her neck, upper back and legs.

In July 2004 Anita felt the herbs were having a consistent enough effect for her to stop taking Methotrexate, which she knew was damaging her. She resolved she could increase her use of Celebrex to help her with any extra pain and at last we could look at some of her true symptoms. We kept adjusting the dosage of her herbal medicines and how often she took them so that she didn't need to increase her daily dose of Celebrex. Still, she was afraid of waking in the morning in agony without the nightly dose of Celebrex. So we created a mixture of herbal medicines and oils to be applied with dressings to her painful joints, and left these on overnight.

Also, in July 2004, we investigated whether flower essences would support the repair of this serious condition of psoriatic arthritis. I used Kinesiology to talk to her body and we muscle-tested from the Bach Flowers, the Himalayan Enhancers and the Humanifest Essences. We asked her body to tell us the best mix to help. Her body wanted a lot in one mix, so we put them all in together.

I made them into a 500 ml mix—the most complex and largest flower essence mix I had ever made! I gave her a 25 ml dropper bottle to decant into from the 500 ml mix so she could carry the mix at all times and take it regularly all day. Over the next six months, it became more and more obvious that if Anita missed taking this flower essence emotional support mix for more than a day her body would react with difficult symptoms which felt to her like going backwards.

These treatments worked so well that by November 2004 Anita felt confident enough to put the Celebrex in the bin. Treatments with the Doctor of Chiropractic had demonstrated with Kinesiology that although Celebrex had an ingredient that helped her problem it also contained something that made her problem worse, most probably one or two of the additives.

Anita felt so good and so in control with her range of supplements and herbal medicines that by November 2005 she wanted to come off the 5 mg daily dose of Prednisone as well. She felt that the psoriasis, which was now nearly covering the whole of her torso, would only get better when she was off all pharmaceutical drugs. She chose to stop it suddenly and see if she could manage the withdrawals with herbs and supplements. Five days later her joints were very swollen and she was in a lot of pain.

The result of this dramatic withdrawal was too much and Anita ended up having to go back on a much higher dose of Prednisone. She went on 10 mg daily and her psoriasis got even worse. She couldn't hide it under clothes any more. It covered the whole of her trunk, front, and back, and was creeping up her neck and down her arms and legs.

Anita's sensitivities didn't decrease and wouldn't for many years. My understanding of this comes from my own body. The pathways that are involved in the long-term development of inflammatory reactions take a long time to repair and the memory in the cells takes many cellular replacements to disappear. Emotional chemical cascades are involved as well as physical damage.

At one stage when her wrists, ankles, and knees swelled up and we couldn't find a reason. I asked her what had changed about her diet. Pausing for just a moment she replied, 'Oh I've been introduced to balsamic vinegar and I love it. I've been having it on my salads every day'. To her disappointment, I had to inform her that many balsamic vinegars have sulphur preservatives in them.

At the end of 2007, Anita was only on 3 mg of Prednisone daily. She was trying a new pharmaceutical medication which was helping her psoriasis. She had no intention of using it for long; it was just to give her extra support to withdraw from the cortisone.

She was working full-time, teaching high school students, which she loved and it nourished her. We were still working on repairing her liver, adrenal glands, and digestive system with herbal mixes.

Her adrenal glands were slowly regaining the ability to produce her anti-inflammatory hormones so that she could slowly tail off the cortisone. She still took her anti-inflammatory pain relief herbs every day—some days only once and some days three or four times. The dose she needed was much lower than two years previously. Anita knew when she needed them.

Her knees were hardly ever swollen and her fingers were no longer bent any more. Her head was straight and moved easily. She did not walk stiffly and she was not in need of knee replacements. Her psoriasis was almost gone. She was proud and graceful again.

At one point, Anita and her partner had to move house during the school holidays and be ready to start work at a different school. Moving in two weeks and starting work certainly made her body pump adrenaline and we discovered that she felt better for this. Three years previously she hardly had the energy to pack a suitcase or get to work. I suggested that the next stage of repair may be an exercise programme at the gym.

I believe the scarlet fever damaged her adrenal glands severely and the anaesthetics for the hip replacement operations increased this damage. The long-term antibiotics for her scarlet fever were needed to save her life, but the sulphur in them was destructive to her system. Also, that they damaged her gut flora (acidophilus, bifido, bulgaricus, and other colonies) which should reside throughout her small and large intestines to assist digestion of food. Without these colonies, we cannot digest food and obtain proper nutrients for healthy functioning and for healthy cell reproduction. No one knew then how important it is to take probiotics while taking antibiotics to re-introduce the necessary gut bacteria.

I also believe the little girl Anita began having digestive problems when her beloved little brother was sick. She remembered how she felt holding him in the night and praying. When I asked for her approval to put her story in this book she sent me a wonderful email, which included this:

> *Also, from my point of view, I feel that you haven't emphasised enough the importance of your support for me during that time. Both through taking the herbs, but also emotionally. In hindsight, the time and care you gave me was as healing as the herbs and supplements. It was such a difficult isolating period of my life and you were 100 per cent on my side, had my*

back and were available for me whenever I needed it. That was incredibly supportive, and I've never had that from any health practitioner before or since then. Sending all my love and appreciation …

She wanted me to warn people about withdrawing from Prednisone—it needs to be really slow because of the danger of adrenal failure, and I would add that if you can find a good herbalist to support you with herbs it will be a little easier—but only reduce by 1 mg at a time every few weeks while your body adjusts. [More details about the herbs and dosages used in this story are detailed in Chapter 24, page 137.]

CHAPTER NINE

The doctor's husband

One day I answered the phone to a very unusual request. On the other end was a doctor I knew from our international herbal medicine conferences. She had also trained to be a herbalist. She said she was calling me because she didn't think she knew enough about herbs to be treating her husband. She had heard that I was brave enough to go into hospitals and treat patients in need of my help.

Her husband was in the Intensive Care Unit (ICU) of a hospital and unconscious with serious pneumonia, contracted while undergoing treatment for quite advanced cancer. The doctors attending him were sure this pneumonia would finish him off because he was very frail.

We talked in detail about his condition and recent medical history which, of course, she was well informed about. I told her I didn't hold much hope of being successful and I didn't believe it was okay to treat an unconscious man. She explained to me that as his wife she was able to make the decision to have the herbal treatment and she intended to be the one to give him my herbal mixes.

I explained that I wouldn't be able to put my label on the bottle because I could get into serious trouble. Also, I believed that he needed at least 5 ml doses of my mix every hour to have any chance of being effective. She said she could manage that.

I said that once I had mixed and blended his medicine I would be removing the alcohol and replacing it with honey and water to avoid giving an unconscious man battling cancer any alcohol, which could be a bit too toxic at such high daily doses. On the phone, she said, 'Great. So please put a blank label on the bottle that says MANUKA HONEY and nothing else written on it. Make it a 500 ml bottle and plan to just leave it with me and I will make sure he gets it'.

Intrigued, I did as she said and drove to the hospital. I was allowed in to see her sitting at the side of her husband in ICU. For each patient in ICU, there was one nurse permanently watching over them. As I arrived the nurse left briefly to fetch the next bottle of liquid food that was being fed into him through a tube straight into his stomach. When he came back the doctor explained to the nurse that she just needed to add some of the Manuka honey her husband's liquid food mix before it was connected it up to the tube system. We had already calculated how many millilitres of the herbs to add to the new bottle of liquid food.

She measured the herbs, added them to the liquid, and replaced the empty container with the new one containing my herb mix. Then she explained it all to the nurse in charge and together they wrote up the instructions on the chart so to help each nurse on duty add the same amount of 'MANUKA HONEY' to each new container of food.

I was nervous. Not about the herbs I had mixed for him but about whether she would get into trouble for doing this. I expressed this to her and she was dismissive. She told me something that day I had never thought about. She told me that the doctors at the hospital would not question her about what she was doing for a few reasons. First and foremost because she was a doctor. Second because if they knew what was in the bottles I had brought in they would have to stop the staff administering the herbs. As soon as they knew, they became legally liable in case the herbs interfered with his treatment. Lastly, because they believed he was dying anyway.

He didn't die though. He got better and went home, came through the cancer treatment and lived for another two years. His wife, the doctor, was happy.

Intriguing to learn that as soon as any treatment other than pharmaceutical was mentioned as a possibility for a patient under their care, the medics would have to stop it as too risky. Some people think it's because they don't know anything about herbs. Which of course they don't.

I had experienced the odd specialist confronting me early on in my practice when they found out I was also treating someone who had become their patient as well. They were derisive about the possibility of me being able to help with herbs. I used to struggle to tell them how many wondrous things my herb mixes could do to help their treatments become more effective. They would often give me their opinion that I really had no evidence to back up my claims. I wasn't rude enough to tell them that they had very little evidence that their medicine could be effective either.

CHAPTER TEN

My brain is eating my pituitary gland — Karen's story

Opening the door to welcome Karen for her first session was a surprise. Her ex-partner was a student of mine, studying herbal medicine at college. He was a young-looking 40-year-old. Before me was a grey, stooped, sad woman. She shuffled and dragged herself up my corridor, sinking into the chair I offered her, and sighing with exhaustion. She was very thin, had too many wrinkles on her yellowy-grey face, and her hair was lifeless. Around her was a cloud of hopelessness.

Karen was 42 years old. I asked her why she was here.

> I've been diagnosed with an autoimmune disease and my pituitary gland is under-functioning. It was diagnosed four years ago and my treatment is a daily low dose of cortisone. I have blood tests every six months to check my thyroid functions. The T3 and T4 are always raised and the growth hormone is low and TSH is low too. My pituitary gland can't produce enough TSH to help the thyroid function better and my blood pressure is always low (90/70). I get constant infections, mostly head colds and sinusitis—maybe because the cortisone suppresses my immune function. I have constant headaches, exhaustion, and stuffy head and I carry a puffer for my asthma that I use one to three times daily.

I asked her why she sought a diagnosis four years ago.

> *I had a major challenge at work and it was affecting me badly so I resigned over it. Straight after I resigned an aggressive thug was sent to escort me out of the building. Almost immediately I developed a very bad sinus infection. The doctor gave me antibiotics, which he kept me on for eight weeks and I still had it, couldn't shake it. So the doctor sent me to an immunologist who sent me on to an endocrinologist. They were checking my auto-immunity. The endocrinologist sent me for an MRI and when I went for the results she told me that an autoimmune problem was in my pituitary gland. She said something was eating away my pituitary gland deep inside my brain.*

Antibiotics for eight weeks can do a lot of damage to the gut. I asked Karen, 'Did the specialist show you the MRI photos while she was telling you this and was there a light behind them? Did she point out your pituitary on the pictures? Did she say what could be eating away your pituitary gland?' She replied, 'I saw the photos but there was no light behind them, just a whiteboard I think. She didn't show me anyone else's. She just said that mine was obviously misshapen and that she'd never seen anything like it'.

I didn't ask her what could be eating at it. I felt so shocked I couldn't say anything. I showed her two photos and one illustration of normal pituitary glands in my medical books and asked her if hers looked the same. She told me that it did: the same as a normal pituitary gland.

I asked her questions about her menstrual cycle which is mainly controlled by the pituitary gland. It had been completely normal, regular as clockwork every 28 days, without pain, until 12 months ago. Then it began to be irregular, about every two months, as well as painful, heavy bleeding and with severe PMT. At the time she thought this was because 'something was eating away my pituitary gland'.

Since corticosteroids should be produced by healthy adrenal glands to serve the needs of the body—such as for anti-inflammatory action or pain relief—I asked if she knew of any reason to believe her adrenal glands weren't functioning well. 'I have arthritic symptoms in my fingers and wrists which started about two years ago and have been getting worse quite fast and I have bursitis on one elbow which is very painful. The doctor has given me two cortisone injections for it but that only helps for a couple of days. Also, I ache all the time from the waist down all the way to the bottom of my feet. My legs feel very heavy'.

Arthritic symptoms come with a toxic liver and digestive problems. Exhaustion comes through having no fuel available in the body. Metabolism of food is controlled by the adrenal glands and the thyroid. Toxic liver comes through ingesting poisonous substances—like antidepressants and too many antibiotics. I asked about her history.

> *I was an only child. My parents drank a lot of alcohol and fought a lot. I was a nervous and anxious child. I had tonsillitis and ear infections from birth until I was six years old and had my tonsils out. Always at the doctor and on antibiotics, according to mum. I remember having terrible gut pain and wind often, from quite young, and having to take laxatives because of the constipation, until I left home. At 25 I was diagnosed with anxiety and panic disorder and given anti-anxiety and antidepressant drugs. I took myself off them when I was 35 and started eating whole foods and avoiding fertilisers, pesticides and food additives.*
>
> *Now I feel like I've got anxiety and panic disorder again. I'm constantly on edge and irritable like I've got PMT all the time. I think it's the destruction going on in my brain, in my pituitary gland. I can't think straight and the headaches just get worse. I don't know what to do. I've been on antidepressants again for three years now and I still feel like this. I have no appetite, I can hardly face eating anything because it makes me feel sick and I'm so exhausted I can hardly stand up in the shower. How I get to work every day is a miracle of willpower.*

I checked my notes with her. 'So you can't eat or digest food easily and you've believed that something was eating away at your pituitary gland and you've been led to believe that because of this you need to be on daily cortisone treatment for four years?' 'Yes'. 'And after a year of being treated for this autoimmune problem in your pituitary you were so distressed you began medication with antidepressants?' 'Yes'. 'And now you have been taking cortisone for four years, Lexipro for three years, and having antibiotics regularly for sinus infections?' 'Yes'.

Together we looked up the side effects of both these medications on the MIMS Online Australia. I knew they were giving her very toxic blood. Then I asked Karen if she'd found anything that made her symptoms noticeably easier.

68 THE MEDICINE WOMAN

> *Actually, I've just finished a course of antibiotics for a sinus infection and for two weeks I have felt better than I've felt for years. Only it feels like I need the treatment for longer 'cause the symptoms are slowly creeping back. The trouble is I got thrush and eczema on the second day of taking the Erythromycin antibiotic and now I have terrible wind and constipation again.*

I put Karen on a diet of Rejuvenex powder and Beyond Greens and some very simple meals. I told her she was to eat five tiny meals a day and to take Tresos B with her first meal of the day. I made her a herbal tonic mix which I designed to be antibacterial, antifungal, antiviral, hormone rebalancing, immune restoring, digestion supporting and blood cleansing. I told her not to take any more antibiotics and asked her to come back two weeks later. She did.

This time I opened the door to a very different person. For a minute I was confused. Karen was a different colour and she bounced up the corridor to my consulting room. She had taken herself off the daily corticosteroid after reading the side effects in the MIMS Australia online. She had followed the diet I recommended, had no sinus problems, and hadn't needed antibiotics.

First I told her about the gut damage that antibiotics do to the gut walls as they strip away the healthy microbes we need to protect our gut walls and to help us digest food. I explained how the gut lining breaks down and allows undigested food molecules to leak through the walls into the bloodstream, which then becomes toxic to the liver. The liver plays a major role in cleaning rubbish out of the blood as the blood makes its way through the liver every 20 seconds to be detoxified.

So Karen knew we had some work to do with herbs to continue detoxing her blood, restoring her liver, cleaning Candida and any nasty bacteria from her gut, and repairing her gut walls. This would improve her ability to digest food. She wanted to talk about how I could help her take herself off the antidepressant tablets. This is not a difficult thing to do with the right herbs. Within three months Karen had no autoimmune problems; a healthy, normal, functioning pituitary gland; and was not on any pharmaceuticals, including antidepressants. And nothing was eating her pituitary gland. This misdiagnosis was another *not* uncommon mistake of specialists.

Pharmaceuticals can help for a while—but every 24 hours the clearance rate of the drugs is only a maximum of 80 per cent, so every day 20 per cent of the drugs are left behind in the body. After two or three months this adds up to a massive level of toxicity and liver overwhelm. Severe depression is the inevitable result. And the side effects start to become overwhelming.

Karen thought, like many people, that a specialist would be someone she could trust. Someone who might know what they were talking about. Instead, she got someone who had no idea, someone making a stab in the dark and terrifying her. This is not uncommon. Even when they are able to diagnose causes, the medics have a very small range of treatments which can be horribly toxic.

SECTION TWO

FINDING THE SHAMAN

CHAPTER ELEVEN

The earth called me

I have never sought out the readings of clairvoyants or medical intuitives. Sometimes they have come to me wanting to offer me their information—their interpretation of the messages that come through them when they stand in my energy field. I bless them for their messages and they always help me feel strong *but*—I'm here now. It's 2024, and in this life I need to be present every day in order to serve for the good of the earth and all life forms.

Guidance from a truth-teller and experienced spiritual healer has been vital—to help me learn discrimination. Clairvoyance is of no use to me. Here are some of their messages and my responses. I ask you to think about how helpful these messages are:

- 'You were Mary Magdalene at the foot of the cross and you are here now to help Jesus come again and to care for him'. *That's a difficult career path!*
- 'You were Joan of Arc's friend, a herbalist, and you made the potion that helped her die before the flames of her death pyre began to torture her'. *Why didn't she listen to me?!*
- 'You have been killed as a witch by many Christian armies and soldiers'. *Men can be so difficult to get on with!*

- 'You are one of the Master Teachers from Sirius who keeps coming back to help humanity'. *I'm tired. I want to go home now!*
- 'You came here with the knowledge of 876 lifetimes as a healer. You came to help humanity remember how they are joined with the earth, how they are dependent on the earth'. *No wonder I'm exhausted. Why aren't they listening?!*

I believe I came to help the plants be valued again. I know that our bodies have such a need for the love of the plants that we long for a healing relationship with them. The healing the plants can do for us happens on so many levels. Try standing inside the aura of a tree, lying in grass that's full of herbs in a field in Norway, rubbing your face into Basil and smelling the release of the fragrance. Try sinking your nose into a real old Rose, *Rosa rugosa*; they were used for medicine in Persia and Ancient Greece. What the smell of that Rose does is to announce to your nervous system that it can heal you on the deepest levels, not just the oil, the whole plant, and not just your spirit, but the *whole* of you: physical, mental, emotional.

My memory is made up of complex dimensions of sensorial experiencing and some of the things I have experienced in this life cannot be presented to you as three-dimensional reality, the kind of factual reality that my friend standing next to me or my father witnessing the child at play may agree is what happened. The reality that I present in this section of my book is my experiential memory—what my senses told me was real at that time.

Now these memories may be coloured by the overlay of stories told to me by witnesses, and language given to me by others; by the use of learned words and through the struggle to be heard and understood. My inability to separate time when I experience the memory in the landscape I walk on means that all time is condensed into that moment, and I am accompanied by the whisperings of the plants that walk beside me.

I was born when the moon was in Capricorn, the planet Uranus was on the horizon and in the constellation of Gemini, and the sun was in Taurus. I didn't cry out loud that I was alive. I moaned and then held my breath to listen. And somewhere nearby I could hear the trees singing.

I am the daughter of a military man, a warrior, and I have that bloodline and that inner strength. And he trained me. With his encouragement and his opposition, with his domination and his trust, with his hypocrisy and his confusion, with his ambition and his misogyny.

It was the time for all of that to be normal. He loved me in his way, and I wasn't going to be normal.

My birth mother was her grandmother's favourite child. She had a special loving soul that people were drawn to and a gift for soothing their pain with love. Her name was Brenda and when she danced with my father people stood back to enjoy the beauty of her. Deeply spiritual, gentle, and kind to everyone, my mother personified grace. Her grandmother had passed on to her a deal of knowledge about the healing herbs of England. My father made her promise not to talk about it and not to talk about her faith.

I crawled early, I climbed early, and I got up and walked at eight and a half months. Soon I headed off to the jungle. I wanted to find the trees I could hear singing. Me and my dog, naked and fearless we explored the edges of the jungle.

I think I remember some of this time. My father's hobby was photography so we have albums of photographs which my family has examined together nostalgically many times. The stories are firmly planted with the words of mum and dad.

As I mentioned earlier, I was taken back to England when I was almost 3 years old where I met my great-grandmother, Ruth, and my nanna, Kathleen, and where I was introduced to the wonders of the trees and plants that would have such an effect on me.

Fast-forward. I was 34 living in Sydney, Australia, when I finished my formal training with my herbal medicine teacher, Dorothy Hall. I already knew it wouldn't be an easy path. My mother died when I was 27, so I lost my spiritual guidance and support, and I'd been warned off herbalism by my grandmother. However, the plants just kept calling me.

At age 36 I felt I needed to find spiritual guidance and teachings. What are the important messages coming from my guides to help me? How do I recognise the messages for me from the angels? In the Adyar bookshop in Sydney, I found a beautiful book called *Crystal Healing* by Edmund Harold. He was living in the Blue Mountains and I contacted him to ask for an aura reading. He picked up the phone and immediately said, 'At last you are here. I've been told to expect you. They said that you are the herbalist who is coming to help me with my healing'.

This was the beginning of a beautiful friendship and learning with this gifted soul. He was an extraordinary teacher who helped his students to find their spiritual gifts and make their connections with guides and angels. These students wanted to take the path of learning to work with spiritual healing. I too wanted this. I believed that choosing to be a herbalist was a crazy, hard path to take.

First, my aura reading with Edmund told me that I have brought the knowledge of healing with herbs from many lifetimes. That I have help available to me from an old monk who accompanies me and a Druid priestess. Edmund told me that these two sit in my aura and are here to guide me. The old monk regularly rolls his eyes upward as if to say, *When will she stop and listen to me?*

Edmund taught me the need to protect myself from trickster spirits bringing false or useless messages, using the Violet Flame around me. He taught me special prayers to help me call for help from my guides or from angels. He said that sometimes souls get caught by their own fears and can't move easily to the light and that these souls can get nasty or play tricks on us—for their own entertainment. That this then can become clairvoyance and is of no use to me. Make sure you only call for help from the light, he told me.

Working with Edmund I learned to sense energies and energy changes; to scan the body with my hands and feel the energy changes. I learned I can see auras if I really concentrate hard, but feeling and sensing them is faster for me. Auras change according to what the person is thinking about.

While I was learning with Edmund Harold he regularly told me that I had no choice about what I would offer people to help them heal. He said it was very clear that I came here in this life to work with herbs; to show people yet again how powerful they are. He told me that people would come to me for help with plants. That is exactly how it happened.

CHAPTER TWELVE

Findhorn and shamanic work

In 2009 I finally went to Findhorn to learn to identify my deepest psychic abilities with Franco Santoro.
Franco wrote the following:

> The term 'shamanism' comes from saman, the Russian transliteration of a word used in Siberia, which means 'somebody who sees in the darkness'. In recent decades the term 'shaman' has been almost universally adopted by anthropologists and mainstream culture to identify people who were previously referred to by other names, such as medicine man, medicine woman, witch, wizard, magician and hundreds of other synonyms.
>
> A shaman is a human being who, out of his will, is able to enter into an altered state of consciousness to relate with realities that are alien to ordinary human beings and use this connection to get wisdom, ecstasy, power, or for healing purposes. In engaging in their activities shamans move between a so-called ordinary state of consciousness and a non-ordinary, or shamanic state of consciousness. In those states the distractions of ordinary reality lessen their pressure on consciousness, making it possible for shamans to focus on the aspects essential to their healing work and reach a condition of spiritual ecstasy or enlightenment. Yet, differing from mystics

> or other advanced beings on the spiritual path, shamans do not aim at enlightenment for its own sake. Their main purpose is that of moving into other realms and then coming back to help and heal their community.
>
> In shamanism, there is no separation and everything is perceived as part of the same unity. The chief trait of shamans is their clear perception of that unity. They are very familiar with states of consciousness that allow visions and explorations of the dimensions that exist beyond the conventional reality. In order to travel to these spaces, shamans use various tools and receive the support of Spirit Guides (also called guardian spirits, power animals, spirit allies, angels, etc).

Franco has written a lot more than this as part of his teachings and in his two wonderful books, *Astroshamanism Book 1, A Journey into the Inner Universe* and *Astroshamanism Book 2, The Voyage through the Zodiac*. Both these books are published by Findhorn Press.

Franco works with us to help us find our soul and feel it. Then he connects us to the Earth and helps us identify and feel all the wonderful ways the Earth is just waiting to help us heal. He leads us in the ways to tune in to our guides and angels, and helps us hear them. He shows us how to tune in and listen and how to put our mind aside and find our sensorial skills.

CHAPTER THIRTEEN

Travelling to Findhorn

I was on my way to Findhorn looking for earth magic and heart healing. Inside me was a longing to lie down on a piece of the world worshipped since 1962 by people connected to angels, devas and earth spirits. A place where plants were grown with such love they thrived on sand and wild sea winds and still became some of the biggest plants the world had ever seen. A place filled with reverence for nature and respect for unseen worlds. I would be there for summer solstice, a time when the twilight of dusk lasts all night and the magic of the misty, shimmering light casts romance and fairies into the air. A time of celebration and communion. I remember it from long ago. The full moon would be huge and so close to the Earth you could almost jump onto it.

In the far north of Scotland, Findhorn is a small point of land just outside the village of Forres on the coast, 30 miles from Inverness. Next stop east, across the sea, is Norway, closer than England. Next stop north, the Arctic Circle and that isn't far away; just a few islands lie between Findhorn and the North Pole. I landed in Inverness, a large town at the mouth of the land where the waves of the Moray Firth carry the legends of the North Sea into the waters of Loch Ness.

I knew I needed a holiday. My work takes me into the suffering minds and bodies of my clients and every so often the responsibilities overwhelm me and my heart weeps. Commonly called exhaustion: nothing left to give. My meditations and my herbal medicines usually maintain me. But the days of living in the city as the planet gets further into crisis are very demanding. The time I get just lying among my plants soaking up their energies is too short. My mind needs some help to switch off, let go and allow physical and spiritual repair.

I searched the net for a retreat somewhere—a silent one. Should I do a Vipassana in India? No, I needed more. On a whim, I checked out the Findhorn website. I found they have a house on Iona, in the Inner Hebrides, where you can go for silent retreats. That was tempting.

Then I looked at what was happening in Findhorn itself. 'The Original Quest: An Astroshamanic Journey into Space and Time ... offering practical tools and understanding for journeying in dimensions beyond conventional time, space ... the programme includes soul retrieval, past life and time voyages, trance dances, rituals'. That's what I needed: to renew my connection with the earth and with the path of my soul.

I investigated the facilitator, Franco Santoro. I'm a bit fed up with the marketing programmes of people claiming possession of shamanic skills. I know a few of them and have heard reports of their workshops. I'm not easily impressed but Franco impressed me. I followed a reference in his online CV and phoned someone who must have been listening to the same master teacher in the late 1970s. I rang them and got only praise for Franco: I made my bookings. The response from Findhorn carried the loving care I wanted.

I got off the plane at Heathrow and onto the train to Luton. Then on a bus to Luton airport, one of England's busiest. Between the station and airport, there were cranes, trucks, buses, tradesmen, shouting—everywhere work in progress. Ongoing expansion in concrete and steel, keeping up with the demands of the travel industry, along with Multi-storey car parks with permanent rooftop building sites adding another storey each year. Endless loops of buses circling the airport to the train station and back, carrying holidaymakers and commuters onto the next stage of their journeys. The airport's main hall was full of people in a hurry, grabbing newspapers to help them keep up with the world.

On the plane I found myself sitting across the aisle from two people chatting about their work at Findhorn. I kept silent and eavesdropped, resolving to follow them at Inverness Airport, and hoped they would lead me to a bus or taxi to Forres or Findhorn. They worked at the Findhorn Foundation, carrying earth healing information and technology out into the world. I wasn't keen enough to *seriously* eavesdrop. I was on holiday and the politics of saving the earth had to be left alone if I was to rest and restore.

I followed them through the baggage collection and outside the airport building. They headed straight for the carpark and I panicked and called out, 'Excuse me, could you please tell me where I can find the bus to Findhorn?' 'Are you going to Findhorn or Cluny College?' the man asked. 'Cluny College?' They looked at each other. 'Come with us. I think we can fit you in the car'. A sparkling redhead at the car welcomed me. 'Of course, we can. I'm Yvonne, this is Martin and this is Jill. You are very welcome'.

I told them my name and then settled into the back seat quietly. Their greetings to each other over, Yvonne glanced in the driving mirror at me. 'Where have you come from and what have you come to Findhorn to do?' 'Sydney, Australia. I'm booked in to do the Astroshamanic retreat with Franco'. Martin, Jill, and Yvonne all smiled. 'Synchronicity', they all said at the same time. Martin followed with, 'I've just got back from Sydney. I've been organising myself an office in Bondi Junction. Where do you live?' 'Bondi Junction!' 'Synchronicity', we said again and laughed. 'And I'm from Sydney too', said Yvonne.

The countryside was hard to see out the side window of the car. I was aware of houses built of dark grey stone and the Highlands in the distance, and when Yvonne called, 'Here's the Moray Firth' I saw a large cove on the left and strained to see Loch Ness on the right but it was too far away.

Twenty minutes later we reached a beautiful village. As we passed the village green Yvonne said, 'This is Forres. I'll show you where we live and if you can find some free time in your retreat schedule I can take you sightseeing. Let's see what Franco wants you all to do'.

'So where is the original Findhorn village?' I asked.

Yvonne answered:

> *Oh, that's the other side of Forres', 'It's now an eco-village and houses the guests who come to learn about creating ecologically friendly housing, villages, and communities. People come from all over the world to attend the workshops held there—architects, and environmental specialists of different kinds'.*
>
> *Cluny House is the spiritual, emotional, and physical healing centre. Workshops and retreats for healing and learning different therapies are*

> held there. About 700 people make up our community, some live at Findhorn and some at Cluny College, and they work and run those places. While you are experiencing your shamanic journey with Franco we have 40 people studying Esalen massage techniques. Other than that it's pretty quiet. During summer we have as many as 1,000 guests here participating in workshops and healing groups.

Then a long tunnel of massive magical guardians wrapped their branches around us and drew us gently up Cluny Hill towards the spiritual retreat. Beech, Pine, Holly, Oak, and Larch trees—an avenue of Bach Flower Remedies. The energy of these trees offers such healing that in 1930 Dr Edward Bach, after testing them for years on his hospital wards full of severely ill patients, created a range of powerful flower essences from the morning dew on their leaves.

Beech is for those whose inner pain drives them to find flaws and imperfections in themselves and others. Pine for the self-reproach of those who feel guilty and unworthy. Holly is for those who are capable of strong love and strong hatred—those who, when negative, get caught in envy, jealousy, revenge, and suspicion. Oak for the dependable, strong, responsible people, to restore them when they crack—because when they fall they become heart-stricken and broken. Larch is for those who lack confidence and feel inferior, so they won't try in case of failure.

Almost all the Bach Remedies grew at Cluny in the garden. So I would be able to drink the morning dew straight off the leaves, and direct it under my tongue, which would send it directly to my brain to rearrange my emotional, chemical, and neuro-cascade whenever I felt the need! The front door was surrounded by Honeysuckle, whose morning flower dew can help release us from the past. I ate a couple of those flowers and then I entered. My whole being relaxed and let go in a deep sigh.

For ten days I ate wonderful whole, organic meals prepared by a team who held hands in a circle and helped each other express and let go of negative emotions before they handled our food. No tortured plants or animals were served there. Our water came in jugs with LOVE written in large letters around the sides. Pieces of cotton lawn edged with beads covered the tops of the jugs and dripped colourfully down the sides of the glass. Fresh flowers were picked daily for each dining table.

In my shamanic work, I became the earth. Every morning I laid down in a patch of Speedwell flowers with English bumble bees buzzing around me and I reconnected with my guides, those old monks who'd been helping me for years. I first met them in my visions while learning from an old spiritual healer who helped me start communicating with them. I laughed to see them shaking their heads at me and wagging their fingers telling me what to get on with next. And my angel came too; one of the group saw him and said he was Michael. Others have seen him and expressed amazement—he's as tall as a house. I don't see him, I feel him, and I feel real safe with him beside me. I cried and cried for all the pain we humans create and spread around. And I got strong again.

That group of 15 people held me and loved me until I was strong enough to come home and work again. And while they held me I felt Claudia's headache and led her to the Feverfew and Lavender calling out to help her. Dave's broken heart followed me and I found Rosemary to help him heal. Jenny brought her grief with me up the spiral hill and we found the morning dew on the Gorse for her to drink. Franco's belly called and together we found Yarrow, Angelica, Sweet Cecily, and Speedwell for him to make a tea, which would take a few months to heal an old digestive struggle and some internal wounds.

Sandra asked me to help her create a ceremony to heal a piece of the garden that was awful to be in. She went to do some research and I went to sit there. I felt terrible pains all over me. Sandra returned from the library to say she found references and drawings in a local history book about the herbalists who were put into wooden barrels with stakes driven through them and their bodies. Then they were rolled down that hill. I made a tea of Comfrey and Nettles, Rosemary, Roses, and Yarrow, and together we led the group in a tea ceremony with healing libations to pour on the earth. As we washed that hill with herbs I heard the priest screeching for their blood and people crying and screaming, 'Witch, witch. Begone!'—and the earth sobbing.

In those ten days, cocooned inside the protection of that house and garden and those caring people, I went to parallel universes, experienced time shifts, communed with bodies and plants and trees, met beings in other dimensions, revisited hidden worlds beyond our senses, astral travelled, and restored my soul and the path of my heart.

CHAPTER FOURTEEN

The train to Scotland

19 March 2010

Departing with sunrise just beginning
I travel over Birmingham—
On the flyovers, we travel in cars and trains.

The future is here and underneath us.
In the dark are wastelands spilling out beyond civilisation,
Small houses squashed among empty crumbling factories.
Hunched, hurrying people,
grey and marching
towards the station for the dawn train.
It's off to work for bank managers and politicians—
to improve profit margins and the GNP no one can eat
to meet the quotas squeezed out of the lives of others.

Birmingham New Street Station at daybreak.
A deserted subway.
One by one
people with blue noses and green-grey drained faces,

squash themselves into the heated lifts
on their way to the main Hall to gather
under the big departures sign.
Bent over in the gloom,
they check for platforms and move along
towards their trains.

Me? I'm waiting for my train to Scotland.
All day I'm on British Rail choofing
along in the beauty of the countryside.
Touching the coast, breezing past the history
of the towns and in between
the Yorkshire Moors, the Lake District, Glasgow.

It's wintry and looks naked now,
this island home of mine.
The trees are sleeping skeletons:
Last year's leaves are rotting beneath and
the sky dour with winter's last snow.
Though small blue gaps promise a wee bit o' sun.

In the hedgerows and on the hills
only firs and pine still wear green.
A few of their neighbours sprout catkins
from their bare branches and
veils of lichen drip damply down.

Waiters with trolleys of hot tea and snacks
travel the aisle back and forth
Sociably.

Suddenly a seat, a park bench, just past Glasgow
on top of a rounded bare hill
looks out from the top of the world.
there—a whitewashed village
with snow-capped mountains behind it.
Water everywhere.

And Pitlochry, entrance to the Cairngorms.
A dark clouds arch over yellow-brown fields.
Grass dead from winter snows.

The silver trunks of birches
shiver and sigh and huddle near streams
that rush and bump and splash over rocks.
White water cascades out of mountain gorges
turning into brooks and rivers,
babbling under stone bridges.
Naked round rolling hills with snow like icing;
melted bits on top picked out by the hungry sun.

Here at last Inverness station,
all white under the snow,
the ticket man chased me onto the train:
'Did you drop this money in the ticket office?'
'Thanks'.

The wonder of Loch Ness and the sea.
A rainbow over the bay welcomes me.
I feel the gravity greater up here
Near the North Pole.

CHAPTER FIFTEEN

The Original Quest with Franco Santoro

I was at a crossroads in my life. There were many paths appearing. I wanted to leave duty and responsibility behind. I wanted to take the path that nourishes my heart. The path of love and joyful service—to offer only what I came this time to give. I wanted to find my original self, retrieve my soul and uncover my sensorial skills, identify them.

In the morning we gathered in our group room to register and meet each other. There were 12 of us and two focalisers, Franco Santoro, the creator of the work we were there to experience, and Sverre Koxvold, the towering Viking gardener, who sailed from Norway 12 years ago, connected, and stayed. Their assistant, Elaine Silverfire, in a cloud of calm, helped us write our personal details down and answer questions. We chatted a little and circled each other, wondering and a little shy. Our group room was above the dining room with a huge bay window looking downhill over the gardens and out to sea.

At lunchtime, we found a table for us with a label on it—'The Original Quest'—and we began uniting over the beautiful food of Findhorn. After lunch, I wandered through the garden and walked into sounds of magic and light from a man playing an instrument like a huge metal gong flat on the ground in front of him. This musical healer ate lunch with me and was now making music like a soft gamelan orchestra. I lay on the grass in front of him and all the cells of my body danced. I was transported to other worlds and other dimensions. His name was Simon.

In the afternoon I entered the group room, seriously, leaving my shoes outside. Inside was a circle of chairs. Straightaway I was the new girl at school again—will I be acceptable, am I normal, who will like me, what should I say about myself so I'm not confronting, what should I not say? I tried to deep-breathe, calm myself, go inside, hold my energy, keep my aura small, and not overwhelm anyone. The circle felt good, the room felt sacred, blessed. I chose my seat in the circle—alone—well away from the two men talking loudly and still with their shoes on. I remember thinking, *They must be new to group work*. The others in the group entered slowly, chattily, beginning to take their seats, choosing carefully who to sit with and where to sit—facing the window, back to the window, facing the door.

The two men chatting were very distracting. I was nervous and easily disturbed. I stood and carefully walked around the outside of the circle to give them helpful advice on how to behave; I crouched down behind and between them: 'I wonder if you could stop talking so loudly, I'm trying to go inside and prepare myself, and by the way you might like to know you should leave your shoes outside the room'. The man on my left was red and tense. 'No I don't want to know and I don't want to leave my shoes outside'. The man on my right slumped and his head dropped forward as though shamed. And I felt immediately that I was his mother. Back in my seat, I was ashamed. I realised I had behaved badly and hurt two people. The German woman I was sharing a room with, Annette, bounced in and sat with me, chatting loudly. I snapped, 'I can't talk to you now. I just told those two guys off for talking'. She looked confused and stopped talking.

Franco arrived in the room rubbing his hands. 'Oh yes, lovely, something strong is going on in here'. He took his seat and introduced himself then asked us all to introduce ourselves and say a few words on where we were from and why we were there. My hands were sweating. This was the bit I was nervous about. I learned the names of the two men—the red, angry one was Dave and the shamed, fair one was Nick. I managed to speak the bare essentials, not really telling them anything about me. I listened. The group started to have shape and flavour.

Franco gave us all a notebook and encouraged us to keep notes. He started to tell us about the work we would be doing there. I knew easily he was a wise and beautiful teacher. His words flowed soothingly through me. He took us into a meditation to help create intentions for our quest. We wrote them down and placed them in a circle around the central candle. More gentle words from Franco, then a meditation to explore which of nature's spaces most nourish us, places we can go to in our imaginations when we need solace. I closed my eyes; I'm looking over the sea, alone in a huge garden.

As I wrote my intention for the week and for my future I felt my guts gurgle and relax with a series of releases:

> *My intention is to reconnect with my deepest self and my path of destiny—to become open in order to receive in relationship and to allow support for writing books so my wisdom and knowledge will help heal the Earth and all living things.*

Break-time and I was in guilt about upsetting Dave and Nick. I made myself a cup of tea and began planning my apology. Taking a seat on a sofa in the lounge I awaited their arrival and my nervousness increased. My cup of tea nearly spilt over as Dave bounded in, jumping over the back of the sofa and landing next to me on my left. 'Wow, you are some strong woman'. Nick followed him, landing on the other side of me, 'You sure are, I'm sticking with you'. I was filled with gratitude instead of feeling rejection, and we laughed our way through my apology. Those guys were clear beautiful souls—no new boys here.

After the break, Franco introduced us to a map of the territory of Cluny Hill College overlaid with a zodiac chart. He gave me new understandings and insights about the energies in the land, and ways of describing what I felt on different parts of Mother Earth. He told us about his search for the central point of Cluny's chart and how he finally found it in the building, just off the entrance reception area. I had felt a kind of vortex when I stood there that evening.

We were to choose one of the zodiac areas to be the territory we worked with during our Quest. Franco offered us his pack of 12 zodiac sun signs and we each drew a card. This gave us an energy to work with for the week. Mine was Libra. I was a little disappointed. I wanted a sign promising more depth and torment to sort through! Never mind, I thought, I've got enough of that to live with in my natal astrology chart. Libra could be just right: harmony, balance, partnership, cooperation, peace. Wonderful. We placed our chosen sun sign card in the circle around the candle in a clockwise order with our written intentions underneath.

Then Franco took us deep inside ourselves to show us how to connect with our guides, how to begin conversations with them, how to invite them to help us, and how to watch for their contact. I felt and saw in the darkness of my third eye, like a vision, a familiar photograph, that old Celtic priest again and the circle of priestesses from long, long, long ago, ready to be with me. *Welcome back,* he says to me, *I'm here always supporting your work.* And those priestesses are an ancient part of my soul. When my longing reaches for them I see myself in the circle dancing and chanting with them. I see myself worshipping the Earth and performing healing rituals with them. I miss them. *We are always with you*, they say. Then why do I feel alone? I cry. I don't know if I am strong enough anymore.

The next morning in our sacred space Franco conducted a baptism/alignment ceremony to align our bodies with our intentions. His drumming and chanting were profound, deep and transformative. He told us that we would spend the mornings in our territory until midday, each day, connecting with our guides, enlisting their support for our intention, looking for answers, watching for ideas on how to support the earth in that territory, and how to repair it. He said we could enlist any of the group we wanted to help us plan and carry out repairs in our territories. Then we set off to meet the territories of Cluny Hill.

We walked through the 12 territories of Cluny, from Aries to Pisces, with Sverre guiding us, feeling the changing energies and seeing what kind of supportive constructions had been made in these territories by people in the past. There were spirals, love benches, underground cells, ponds, teahouses, a Buddha in a meditation grove, carefully placed crystals, and on the power point of the garden a spiral walk with ritual stone circles on the top. We explored ideas and feelings about healing different areas. Sverre told us which places he felt might need a little help by sharing stories from his years of loving the garden. He asked that we communicate to him any ideas we had so the garden and all lifeforms there could benefit.

The afternoon tea break was filled with excitement, creativity, feelings, and connection. Back in our group room Franco's words softly fed my heart and then he sent us outside again to find a tree companion to meditate with in order to imprint each other energetically. This tree would then be ready to support me whenever I called. My tree was a massive Beech at the bottom of the steps on the hillside looking over the central lower garden, towards the sea. I stood in the aura of this ancient lifeform, among the big roots reaching down into the Earth, with the blue Speedwell flowers all around, and felt that ancient strength seeping into me.

Next, it was time to get to know my territory. The building part of the Libra sector included the guest reception, the smoker's lounge, the toilets, the ballroom, the tennis court which is now a car park, the entrance to the car park, the small pavilion, and the woods behind it. I looked all around but couldn't find a single thing wrong or that needed changing. In this beautiful area, my territory for this quest, I saw that I had open space to welcome visitors. They could park and stay and play and find privacy and shelter from storms in the pavilion; I could walk with secret lovers in the woods; I could cleanse and release in the toilets and go dancing in the ballroom.

I found my spot to meditate. In front of the pavilion, where lovers once met secretly, and under the two Lime trees, I lay down on a slope in a bed of soft grass. Around me, the grass was filled with the violet-blue flowers of Speedwell and visiting bumble bees heavy with pollen. Alone on my left, the anxious Aspen tree quivered even though the breeze was only slight, and on my right the four baby Silver birches huddled and whispered to us, *We are all safe here*.

I saw beds of Lady's mantle offering their cloak-like leaves for medicine to wrap around and strengthen female parts and the tissues of the lower body, with Yarrow and Nettles to assist; Red poppies with juicy seed pods to calm the heart and help relax and sleep. I saw Ribwort to soothe and rejuvenate lungs and kidneys, restoring lifeforce and the ability to breathe deeply. I saw Wood betony offering to soothe the liver and calm the nervous system—reducing the headaches that can come from deep inner tension and the toxicity of the world. And on the border between my Libra territory and Andrea's Scorpio territory was a Holly tree, whose morning dew waited to help humankind let go of self-hatred, hatred, and desire for revenge.

With Franco, I began to recognise how I experienced the fourth dimension and I learned how to go there with ease. I learned that regular recapitulation is needed—that means scanning for and releasing old memories that give a stuck energy and which can contribute to illness. He taught me the past belongs to the web of life—it is not mine—it belongs to the collective. New intentions need energy, so clearing out memories leaves space for new life. And during recapitulation, no interpretation or analysis is necessary or helpful; this can make the clearing more difficult.

We, the group, began drawing our spiral of life to find the damage that hadn't been cleared which may stand in the way of our new intentions.

We overlaid it onto the zodiac of Cluny Hill and mine was in Capricorn. What a surprise! My moon is in Capricorn in the seventh house, the Libra house of relationships. I went to Capricorn territory to release this damage and offer it back to the Earth. To find the right place I climbed up behind the pool with the hidden crystals placed in Aquarian territory. Nick was there and his energy supported my determination. As I went on, the trees became thicker and darker and the hill got harder to climb. I found an old heavy steel bunker, the kind used for shelter from bombs falling during the war. This one was sinking into the Earth and covered in rusty holes with dangerous-looking broken pieces sticking out ready to wound an unobservant person. I sobbed with relief for the earth's willingness to take this congestion from me and looked up and saw a Holly tree in the shade, still with dew on the leaves. I drank this healing dew and felt my anger fall away into the earth. A Crab apple tree nearby beckoned and I ate some flowers to help me release the deepest toxic parts of my damage.

All around me, I found Pine, Oak, Rowan, Laurel, Maple, Willow, and Beech. Walking up towards the sunlight I ate a small piece of everything that offered help and bowed my head in gratitude to the plants. Looking around I found myself inside the power point spiral which spanned the territories of Sagittarius and Capricorn. Staying inside the spiral I saw Gorse bushes guiding my way. Reaching the sun at the top I saw flowering Honeysuckle to help me let go of the past and give the darkness inside me back to the Earth.

I sat for a while in the sacred circle of stones on the top of the power hill feeling into the lightness of myself. I called back my soul on that spiral path, and cleared the way in between. When I was ready I went back to my Libra territory and accepted a leaf from the Aspen tree to help clear any anxiety left around the path ahead for me.

After this recapitulation, we all gathered quietly for a walk around the whole territory from Aries to Pisces. Led by Sverre, we offered our pain back into the Earth to add to her compost to enrich the future. On the way I sipped from Rose petals in rainwater, drink of the goddesses, and ate all the leaves that called to me—*Take me, I can heal you, I can support you, I can give you strength.* I ate Dandelion leaves to restore my digestion and clear the tears of my liver; Self Heal to take away the heat of angry disappointments and help me focus my passion; Agrimony to take away the worry; Borage to give me courage; Comfrey to make me stand strong; Angelica to keep me connected to the angels.

CHAPTER SIXTEEN

Flowers: a gift of love from the earth

When my son was 3 years old he and I were driving away from the property where he was born. He was in the back strapped into his child safety seat. He had his arm trailing out the window brushing plants as we passed them. Suddenly he screamed and I looked back to see his arm had been slashed open just above the elbow and blood was pouring out. This was scaring him. I couldn't stop the car fast enough to help so I spoke loudly and calmly as I was stopping the car and finding the Rescue Remedy;

'Stop now, look at your arm, and think hard about stopping that blood, pull that blood back inside your arm. You can do this'. I got out of the car and hurried round to his side of the car. He was very focused on the wound. He said, 'Look, Mum, I can do it!' I was amazed. Sure enough, he had done it. We didn't need the Rescue Remedy. I said to him, 'Well done. You keep that blood inside your arm and I can put some healing cream on it just as soon as we get through this gate'. That was the beginning of him learning how powerful his mind can be.

Still, we used Rescue Remedy often to prevent shock and trauma from distorting cells after accidents. We always used it on the site of injuries to the body *and* in the mouth so that the trauma didn't stay in the brain and nervous system.

Years later I was in my healing studio at the end of my herb garden mixing medicines when I bumped myself hard against the pointed corner of a table, straight into my upper thigh. As the pain started I found myself yelling and reeling with the shock, looking around for the Rescue Remedy.

Then I remembered I had left it up at the house. So I stopped shouting in pain and said to myself, 'Pull yourself together, you can send the energy of Rescue Remedy straight down to your injury and the pain will stop immediately'. I concentrated on taking the RR energetic profile from my mouth to my leg and the pain stopped, and the bruising was stopped in its tracks. No more pain, no bruising, no damage.

Edward Bach was a well-respected Harley Street Doctor and the Registrar of a big hospital in London. Not a well man himself he used to travel to the countryside regularly and walk among flowers and forests. This is how he discovered that the morning dew from flowers could dissolve emotional pain or harmonise character traits that had a negative impact. He started to use the remedies on his patients, as he discovered that these negative emotional states were part of causing illnesses like TB to remain with the patient. The stuck emotions were preventing their recovery from serious illness.

Edward Bach compared these patients to the ones who recovered and noted that the ones who recovered were the ones who could drop the stuck emotions or painful thoughts. I call them sabotage programmes. Letting them go, shifting them, and choosing to make new pathways of thinking are all more modern ways of describing this. He began to write up his experiments and resulting theories in the medical journals of his day (around 1930) and doctors from all over the world began flooding in to his talks. That is until someone negative from modern medicine began sabotaging him and his ideas …

Nevertheless, he happily left modern medicine and took up a job as Administrator of the London Homoeopathic Hospital. His Bach Flower Remedies, including Rescue Remedy, are still famous; still used with great success; and still ridiculed by Medical Associations in the UK, US, and Australia, despite nearly 100 years of patients successfully using them and claiming to benefit. It requires an amazing determination to ignore the patient's own feedback, and to hang on to critical thought instead of listening to human reports.

In 2002 I heard that my old friend David Parsons had finally returned from India where he had been living in Osho's Ashram in

Pune for over 20 years. We were friends at University in Adelaide in the early 1970s. Another old friend sent me David's email address. I emailed him and he straightaway answered and invited me to come visit him in Tilba Tilba on the south coast of NSW. His spiritual name is Tanmaya. He had become a massage therapist and energy healer in the Ashram and after Osho passed away he wandered off to the Valley of the Flowers in the Himalayas and began to make vibrational healing flower essences.

I drove straight down to his place and found we had years of talking still to do and we'd grown with the same fascinations—healing with plants and vibrational remedies, listening deeply to patients. We started talking and we still are absorbed by sharing insights and bodily and emotional knowledge and experience. I learn so much from his experience with meditation and subtle energies. He quickly became one of my best teachers and his ability to express how he feels emotionally and how his body feels physically makes him one of my best and most interesting patients.

He is a gardener and has created a flower paradise around his place on the side of Gulaga Mountain. I helped him add many medicinal herbs and taught him how to make his own medicines from them. He sent me home after that first visit with the entire set of his Flower Enhancers and has taught me how to use them. When I display them in my consulting room everyone wants some.

Since I had them to use I hardly even think about using Bach Flower Remedies. I feel that Bach's wonderful range is a little dated and that our emotional world has become so much more complicated since the 1930s. It doesn't mean they don't work in so many good ways, but for me and my patients I like the Himalayan Flower Enhancers.

I really like the way Tanny makes them which is different to how Bach made his. He says his are not 'remedies' because humanity doesn't need remedying but often needs 'enhancing'. I have seen them have immediate and powerful effects on a person, and experienced it for myself too.

In 2009 Tanny went to visit the old-growth forests in Tasmania and met many mushrooms there. After he returned home he dreamed the mushrooms were calling him to make essences with them. He packed up his kit and off he went with a friend to help him. The range is called Tasmanian Wilderness Essences. Seems like they work on past-life ancestral healing. Tanny doesn't work that out himself; he listens to the mushroom and then gives the essences to a whole range of sensitive people he knows and gets their feedback over quite a few years.

One unique thing about flower essence makers is that they all talk about flowers talking to them—guiding them on how to help humanity with them. I travelled with Tanny to the Isle of Gigha in the Inner Hebrides to attend an International Flower Essence Conference. It was such an inspirational and amazing event. Essence makers from Argentina, Alaska, California, Yorkshire, and Gloucestershire, all totally in love with flowers and all walking alone around the mansion gardens on Gigha in the early morning, talking and listening to flowers. Their talks and slide shows were spectacular. Their dining room conversations were somewhat crazy but quite stimulating and entertaining.

In January 2003, my friend Wendi Forbes of Humanifest Essences called me up and invited me to come with her the following evening to an area of the Blue Mountains where one of the world's rarest flowers had been spotted.

The next night was the January full moon in Leo and Wendi was called to make a flower essence with the Pink flannel flower we would find there. She said to bring a bottle of magic special water, a beautiful bowl, my meditation cushion, my camera, a warm shawl, a magnifying glass, and some scissors.

Wendi arrived to collect me before dusk and off we went. She told me that these flowers only grow after the worst kind of bushfire, a fire so vicious that nothing is able to grow there for well over a year. The following spring, after the fire, enough rain comes to soak the ground just at the right time for the flowers to wake up and pop out. They are known to only appear every 50 years. We may only have one chance in our lifetime to see these flowers. And they stay for only two days before they disappear back into the earth.

We found somewhere to park the car. We walked through some bush and out onto an overhanging clifftop just as the full moon was rising over the deep valley ahead. That moon was huge and looked close enough to touch. The scene was eerily strange. All the burnt tree stumps were black and dead-looking with no new growth at all. The moon showed us the area was filled with small bushes covered in exquisite pink flowers. Wendi has a photo of me bent double with my magnifying glass examining the most beautiful flowers I have ever seen. She told me to find a place to sit in meditation with my bowl of magic water and to cut some flowers so they dropped onto the water and floated.

Finding a place to sit wasn't easy because the bushes were all quite close together and I didn't want to squash any. Finally, I found a place to squeeze into and settled myself with no idea where Wendi had found her sitting place. In the full moon peace of that strange landscape, I finally experienced flowers talking to me. They were so happy to have us there making essences with them for healing humanity. These flowers came for humans who had suffered such devastation that they needed these essences to help them begin recovering. They wanted to be helping people to make connections with each other—to dance together and to love again. I cried with joy that night, sitting within the manifestation of the glory the flowers brought to heal the earth and humanity.

I only needed to pick a few to make a powerful essence but I cut as many as they told me to. I didn't want to go home that night and miss any second of that joyous experience. When the time came for me to go it was clear the Pink flannel flowers were telling me to go home and finish the preparation of the essence. Then Wendi appeared and it looked as though she had been sent off by the flowers at the same time.

* * *

In the Australian summer of 2015, my dear friend Ses Salmond came to stay to make medicines with me from my medicine garden. It was a full moon weekend and in the soft dusk of the evening, we were coming across the veranda to the front door, between the sweet-smelling large Daphne bush and the Ginger flowers that love to pump out their scent at night, with our bunches of medicinal herbs to make medicines in the evening. As we passed the Ginger the full moon was high enough in the sky to be lighting up the flowers. They were calling out to become a flower essence so I asked Ses if she wanted to help me make a full moon flower essence with them. Of course, she did.

We prepared a bowl of the energised special spring water I always had at home for making medicines and we put it in a magic pottery bowl made for me by a patient who was a potter. Then we took it out onto a table on my front veranda and said some prayers and thanks to the goddess of the moon and to the flowers. Then we cut some of the Ginger flowers and left them out in the front garden under the moon to help them infuse their energy into the water.

In the morning we bottled the essence water and called it Full Moon Ginger Essence and got on with making herbal medicines.

At mid-morning tea break, we looked into the big bowl wondering what to do with the essence water left over. I scooped up two mugfuls of it and said I thought we could have a mug each. We happily and gratefully slowly drank the new flower essence, and contemplated what it could be doing to us as we drank.

We spoke slowly, almost at the same time, or expanding on each other's descriptions. The following is what we experienced: head clearing—letting go of any tension-making thoughts which made letting go of upper-body tension happen—heartwarming and expansion of the heart—energy flowing down through our legs and Earthing us. At the same time, we experienced the third eye opening—feeling blocked channels opening in the body and clearing—making us both smile to be experiencing the discovery of our own beauty—lung energy expanding so we could take in life more fully—anxieties about the future disappearing; and I can't remember which of us said it but I know we both began to laugh as one of us said, 'Goodness me, I think I can fly'.

Years later at an Aboriginal Women's Healing weekend that Ses organised and I helped her with, we were telling the women about making flower essences and we told them this story on the second night around the fire. One of the native women with us topped off our story with: 'That's what two mad white naturopaths do to have a good time!'

They all came out with us the next morning to make flower essences on the banks of the Colo River on the tribal lands of the Boorooberongal clan of the Darug people. Yarramundi was their herbalist doctor and the Elder recognised by the white invaders as their chief. It was his spirit that guarded the place we were in for those three days of healing that we all came together for. And it was his spirit that was called on to give us permission to take pieces of the land and plants there to make our Yarramundi healing essence. We all experienced it before we went home and everyone took a bottle of it with them after they helped me bottle it into fifty-two 50 ml bottles.

CHAPTER SEVENTEEN

Memories in the land

During my young years, I experienced visions in a number of places that were either historical temple ruins or holy places. These sites were in Cyprus at the Sanctuary of Aphrodite (a place of pilgrimage in the Ancient World for centuries); in Paphos near where the goddess was known to have risen from the sea to create the world; in Cappadocia, Turkey, in a city carved out of the inside of a mountain to be a hidden refuge for Christians escaping from the Romans; in Jerusalem, within the old city walls; at Fountains Abbey in North Yorkshire, UK; at a deserted Stonehenge in Wiltshire, UK; and many other locations especially those local to where I grew up in the UK and in countries around the Mediterranean.

My visions were sometimes like small movies, always behind closed eyes or in the dark. The thought crossed my mind that they might be memories of past lives. I dismissed that idea as useless to me. At one stage I believed they came from cellular memory—which I still think is a possibility, but still not a useful idea to ponder on. My focus is that I am here now and I have work to do.

Years later I came to Australia and learned about Aboriginal peoples' spiritual beliefs about the land as a living, breathing being and their connection to ancestry through place. And my visions still came—in sacred Aboriginal places.

On 11 November 2011, I headed off with my friend Riki to visit Aboriginal Rock just outside Wentworth Falls in the Blue Mountains. Astrological reports told of a portal between worlds and time zones that would be accessible at 11 am. Riki wanted to sit in the cave below the rock. Aboriginal paintings are on the walls of the cave.

We came to the rock and I was drawn to lie down on it. It was a clear day and sunny. Riki left me there and went towards the cave entrance on a level below us. As I lay there I closed my eyes. Clouds gathered, thunder rumbled, and rain began to fall; I could hear it. I opened my eyes and a large hole in the clouds above me seemed to be leaving a space around me where no rain fell. I closed my eyes again and a light like a follow spot beam (spotlight) shone down on me strongly and a voice spoke to me, telling me to believe that I had been given my life to remind people about the herbs they need to connect with and use again.

I was shown visions of past lives I'd had. And the power of that light came into me and healed my soul. When I opened my eyes the clouds had all gone and Riki was quietly sitting nearby, waiting. Everything around me was soaked but I was quite dry.

Riki said that she had come back to the rock twice. The first time I was not there lying on the rock so she went back to the cave. The rain had been heavy and, according to her watch, she had first left me lying on Aboriginal Rock well over an hour ago. I was pretty sure I had not walked away from the rock and neither of us could work out why I was completely dry. Aboriginal Rock is a sacred portal for the transmission of messages or time travel.

* * *

In 1992, I travelled with the Page brothers (Stephen, Russell, and David) and two other dancers to the Northern Territory. I was their Production Manager for a theatrical tour they had created to take to the main theatres in Darwin, Alice Springs, and Adelaide. Although I was already practising as a herbalist, I had been a Production Manager in theatre, opera, music, and dance for ten years previously so my work history was known to a few people in the arts world. Their attitude to my new career path was 'Let us know when you want to come back to work'. One of them offered me the job and told me the three Page brothers were about to be given a grant to form the first Aboriginal dance company in Australia.

The brothers were extraordinarily talented wonderful people. I was very excited and really there was nothing else that would have tempted me—I had worked in London and Sydney on some of the most famous shows of the 1970s. So I happily took the job and found myself sitting in the rehearsal room with these three brothers creating the dance and music for a show that would be the first Aboriginal dancing to be introduced to the broader public of Australia and overseas.

They were all dancers but David was also a 'songman'. Watching Russell dance was like watching liquid silk; Stephen was the dancer/choreographer and an awesome creative leader. I call him a speaker/politician/leader of his people. I mean politician in the finest sense of that word. He became the first Aboriginal Artistic Director of the Adelaide Festival of Arts, and a Film Director, showing the way for his people to step into creative roles in television, film, acting, and writing.

The history of the Bangarra Dance Company is well documented now, as well as Stephen's pathway to help his people step out of oppression, show us how amazing their ancient culture is, and reveal to us the pain they have suffered in modern Aboriginal history. What a leader he is.

Back to our tour together. In that rehearsal room, they created a show full of emotion that tore my heart to pieces. I used a lot of tissues. Russell started the move to come and sit with me if he had strained a muscle or had twisted something. He used to say: 'Can you put your hands on this for me, tidda? I need your healing'. 'Tidda' means 'sister'. Russell told the others I was a medicine woman. After that they all three just came with their hurts and sat with me, placing my hands on where it hurt. They said it made them better. I loved them.

When the show was on in Alice Springs they borrowed the Arts Council bus on the Sunday then came and got me. They said they were taking me on a special trip to Uluru. They told me to sleep on the back seat because I needed some rest.

I did that until I woke up with the small bus slowing to a halt. *Oh dear—we've run out of petrol*. I must have looked very panicked. The road from Alice Springs to Uluru is 454 km and takes four and a half hours to drive. It is dead straight, running through totally flat desert land, with hardly any traffic to be seen on an all-day drive. Stephen piped up, 'Don't worry, tidda, we have a petrol can in the back. I'll be able to go get some petrol and be back soon. Won't take me long time'. And off he went.

As soon as he stepped out of the bus a car came along, picked him up and flew off with him. There were no petrol stations between Alice Springs and Uluru. The others got out of the bus and danced. I went straight to sleep again believing it could be a couple of days before we would be moving along again. Never mind, we had brought a packed lunch! Within the hour another car heading for Alice Springs dropped Stephen back to us with two full petrol cans. Magic, I reckon.

Arriving at Uluru was very special—a rare event. It was raining and the whole of the massive rock was a waterfall with colour-filled bouncing rainbows streaming down with the water. We all stood there and worshipped this huge rock rising up out of flat land all around it—the spiritual birthplace of all life—all songlines—some say the heart chakra of the world.

David Page, my dear friend the song man, standing next to me, said: 'Look at this, tidda, Uluru is offering to make us magic. If we take our clothes off and jump in the water we become magic. Let's do it'. Of course, I did it. We all did it. It was magic. *They* were magic.

Before we got back to Sydney we were notified that they had been given the grant to create the Bangarra Dance Company. They asked me to stay with them and help train their people to become their own Production Managers. I was so tempted but I had a 9-year-old son staying with his grandfather so that I could work with them on a tour, and he needed me at home with him. His father had left—well, I asked him to leave. And I was on the verge of moving to the Blue Mountains and being a medicine woman.

David came regularly to stay with me in the mountains, sometimes bringing his mother, or Russell, or a sister, when they needed help from my medicine. David and I had a very strong connection so we kept on talking regularly and they kept me a ticket for every show for 30 years—I sat with the family.

Eight years later they brought their people from all over Australia to perform at the Sydney Olympics. David created the music, Stephen choreographed, and Russell led the dancers. It was a massive gathering of tribes from all over Australia who answered Stephen's call and an awesome appearance and display of indigenous tribes and people. Thank you, spectacular Page brothers! You have infected the world with love and laughter. You have shared with us your magic.

CHAPTER EIGHTEEN

My Chamomile and Lavender cloak

My first journey to the underworld, I believe, was in dreams and prayers spoken aloud when I knew sometimes that my mother was close to death and that she wasn't going to live for as long as I wanted her around. Her connection to the spirit world was strong and her love was a palpable force that kept us travelling safely in 'the real world'. When I dreamed she was drowning and I couldn't save her, I would wake up screaming but she was always there beside me. This dream was a repeating dream throughout my early life. My sister dreamed regularly that my mother was falling to her death.

We were always loved and secure with her. After she died my sister's dream stopped but mine did not. It happened less often but my dream turned into a visit from my mother. She would come out of the water and talk to me—sometimes just holding me and telling me she was with me and working with my guides. My sister sometimes gets messages from her during times of being awake.

While I was living and working in London, I had dreams and nightmares before she had a brain haemorrhage, and then more during the time she had a huge operation until she gave up and went into a coma before slipping away. In my dreams, I spoke to her in the coma.

I tried to call her back. She didn't want to come back and be a burden to us. She told me I would always be able to reach her. It took her three weeks to die. I wrote all my dreams down at the time. They are like a horror story.

I first consciously went on a journey to the underworld with Edmund Harold and then with Franco Santoro. I was taken on a guided journey that lasted two days with Glynn Braddy in Sydney. I was always given a cloak of Chamomile flowers intertwined with Lavender and was seated on a throne made of a massive old tree with branches that cradled me. I was there to be introduced to my knowledge and strength and the love of the trees and flowers. The cloak was always put on my shoulders by my mother and grandmother and great-grandmother.

These days I often wake up through a hazy smell of Chamomile and Lavender and I know my friends the plants are with me. Sometimes I long to be able to knit this cloak for myself so I can be finally laid to rest in it. I can't rest yet—I have a granddaughter who looks like becoming my apprentice and I have gifted students I need to keep teaching.

I never send a patient home with a mix of herbs or flowers—I never have. I tell them I need to meditate on the best mix for them. In the early days, it was because I wanted to make sure by researching that I was making the very best mix for them. I learned slowly over the first ten years of practice that it was because I was checking the possibilities through my heart-brain and connecting with their deepest physical and emotional disturbances. I know now it is because I can travel through their energy fields and check out where they need the most help—which organ, system, and 'sabotage programmes' need help.

SECTION THREE

THE ART OF PRESCRIBING, MIXING, AND DOSING WITH HERBAL TINCTURES

CHAPTER NINETEEN

How to start

How do we calculate how many drops or millilitres of a herb mix are needed daily by each of our patients?

How many times daily I recommend taking doses depends on the condition of the patient and my diagnosis of the causes; on whether the condition is acute or chronic; on whether we want fast results or slow, gentle, building, or repair. Your patient's progress depends on the strength of each herb in the mix; how strong or weak is their constitution or their current condition; how much stress is around them in their lives; and how long they have had the symptoms or illness. Last but not least it depends on the daily life of your patient and how often they can easily manage to take their doses.

The skill of effective dosing with herbal medicines is the really creative work of a herbalist and this is not learned in a classroom. It is learned from an experienced herbalist and from each patient and their feedback. I believe we need to be considered and gentle with our treatments. We must be cautious and avoid pushing the patient's body out of balance in another way with doses that are too stimulating or with strong alterative herbs like Goldenseal (*Hydrastis canadensis*), Garlic (*Allium sativa*), and Poke root (*Phytolacca americana*). We need to mix these strong herbs with supportive, gentle, tonic herbs to soften their effects.

My dosing recommendations, or instructions, may need to be different for each patient, for each mix used, and the practitioner needs to take into account the energetics of the herb tinctures in the mix. The quality and content of medicinally active ingredients, the amounts of vitamins, minerals, amino acids, and other nutrients will be different in medicines manufactured by different systems of extraction.

We know that all of the ingredients work together to make a herb medicine effective—not just the alkaloids, anthraquinones and glycosides, although these are known as the active ingredients. All the ingredients are important. The vitamins, minerals, amino acids, antioxidants, polyphenols, and enzymes are just as important. They all work together.

Also vitally important are the methods used by the farmers to grow the plant, harvest the plant, dry the plant material; then how long it takes to dry before it is handed over to the manufacturers. We know that as soon as a plant is picked the ingredients begin to diminish. We know this from the research done in the field of nutrition and the testing of nutritional values in fresh foods and dry foods. This is known as the vitality.

Then we have the synergy of herbs mixed together for their combined effect to be increased. A simple example of this is to use an antifungal/antiparasitic/antibacterial herb for a patient with an infection; then add a herb that will support the immune system to produce white blood cells and antibodies to help fight the infection; and then another herb that will keep the lymph glands moving to clear out the dead cells. When you consider the help that the organs and systems of a patient need, there are always other herbs to be added. I usually end up with 11 herbs in my mixes.

We know that Traditional Chinese herbal medicine uses dried plant material and sometimes it seems we don't know how long they have been dried and stored. The mixture in the packet of dried herbs prescribed for you by a Chinese herbalist has to be boiled in water for a few hours before you drink it. Mostly when I boiled my packets of Chinese herbs I had to add four cups and simmer gently until the amount of water was reduced to one cup. This often took three hours on the stove in a Chinese pottery teapot.

The effective strength of the liquid subsequently poured out has not been in question for thousands of years. So we see that heat does not damage this strength. The effectiveness of a brew of dried Chinese herbs once brought me very quickly out of a serious infection of glandular fever.

I was still studying and I had a 2-year-old and no help available. I was worn out and felt quite desperate. All the doctor did was to send a blood test off to pathology and give me the diagnosis. He told me to rest.

A friend recommended I go to a particular Chinese herbalist who worked out the back of a Chinese grocery in Sydney's Chinatown. She told me to go as early in the daytime as I could manage because the queue for his help got longer and longer as the day went on. She said he couldn't speak English very well but not to worry, he would help me. I learned so much going through this treatment.

At the shop, I was given a ticket and shown where the queue was. There were still some seats available. I sat with Chinese people who all had a number on a ticket. I watched each in turn go into a small office with an open door when we heard the man inside call out the next number. No one was in there very long.

This wonderful old Chinese doctor in Sydney's Chinatown felt the pulses in my wrist, and examined my tongue, and chuckled. He wrote my prescription in Chinese and then he tore my prescription off the pad and gave it to me, waved me out of his room to the front desk.

I followed the path of the other patients and found myself in front of a large desk with a middle-aged man behind it. Behind him was a tall and wide chest of drawers with many small drawers in it.

This old and experienced Chinese herbalist became my preferred doctor and treated me whenever I needed help. He used to write sometimes as many as 25 herbs on my prescriptions. He and his son, who weighed up and dispensed the herbs at the front of the shop, helped me learn and understand a lot about the synergism of skilful blending for the symptoms and energetics. The son spoke good English and was happy to answer any of my questions whenever I went for help. He too was a herbalist, and the apprentice to his father.

The dose the old Chinese doctor recommended for me was one mug (brewed as described above) once daily. On that first occasion, it was hard for me to drink a whole mug. I had to work hard to help my stomach keep it down! That took a couple of minutes and then my body just sang and rejoiced and filled up with incredible strength. If I was dealing with acute symptoms I had to go back and be checked and get another prescription, just in case the force and strength of any of the herbs in the mix unbalanced my body in another way.

As I got better and better I would be given a herb mix to take for longer and longer. Very interesting. My serious glandular fever was over in just a few hours after my first dose and two weeks later I was fine again with no post-viral syndrome or chronic fatigue. The Western medicine doctor had told me I would need six weeks of total rest and I had been sick for two months when I saw him.

This was a hard act to follow.

Thus I began to understand that if I wanted to put more than five herbs in a mix for my patients it would not mean I had missed the point, as some teachers try to tell us, but that I wanted a mix designed to support the complexity of the particular patient's body, and the causes, as I understood them, to manage the changes needed to restore health.

I started my practice in 1985 with a range of Nature Spirit 1:8 herbal tinctures making mixes of five herbs in 100 ml bottles and with doses of 25 drops to take between two to eight times daily, depending on whether the symptoms were acute or chronic. I was also determined to make sure that my herb mixes in the first two weeks would heal any pain or distress reported by that patient. I knew that this meant my mixes had to be right and my doses had to work.

This determination of mine meant that at first I was nervous and I refused to send my patients away with their mixes straight after their consultation. I wanted time to think carefully. I told them this and said that I would call them when the mix was ready and we would then arrange pick up or posting. My patients were so happy about this that I never changed this in 39 years of clinical practice. I meditated on the patients, on their struggles in life, and on the best mixes I could make for them. I handed over the mixes along with handwritten dietary recommendations. And I rang them two weeks later to make sure the mixes were working as I had planned and hoped. If the patient wasn't feeling the herbs working, then I changed the doses. Or changed the amount of times a day they should take their herbs. If I changed something then I had to call them again after another week to make sure I had it right.

This is how I learned so much about dosing. This is how I knew when they needed a new mix and when to call the patient back in—by keeping in touch with them. If I knew the herbs were working well I made them a repeat mix to collect. Sometimes I tweaked the next mix with changes designed to make it more effective. I called them again after four to six weeks. When I thought they were ready I told them to take a week off when they finished their current mix and to please let me know if any symptoms returned in case they needed another mix, to make sure the problems had been resolved and repaired. I also gave them some idea of when and why they might need to see me next.

Slowly, by staying in communication with my patient, I learned more about mixing and how herbs in a mix will work together, supporting, restoring, and energising. About what a body can do with herbs. About the synergy of blending. About the magic and alchemy of healing plants. And about the energy of connection, communication and intent between patient and practitioner.

CHAPTER TWENTY

In the consultation room

In the consultation room, we need our traditional philosophies and the knowledge of the effective qualities of our herbs. This knowledge guides us in our questioning of the patient. The philosophies assist us to understand how the patterns of dis-ease begin and progress in the organs and systems of the human body. They help us to diagnose causes, not simply as medical names for conditions of dysfunction, but as disharmonies and imbalances in the constitutions and body systems of individuals who come to us in the hope of finding help.

This is where we start—in the consultation room. How do we assess the patient and where they need help to rebalance and restore their health? Do we use iridology? A great tool to back up our diagnostic skills. Do we use tongue diagnosis? We used to and Traditional Chinese medicine can teach us a lot about this. Do we check the pulses in the wrist? Wonderful for diagnosing disharmony in the systems through feeling and comparing the energies in the body meridians. Do we know how to question the patient about the symptoms? And have we been taught to recognise that certain symptoms give us clues as to, for example, liver malfunctions—so then we ask questions about other liver functions. We don't just stab in the dark and give out St Mary's thistle (*Silybum marianum*).

I was teaching clinical practice to a group of fourth-year Bachelor of Herbal Medicine (B. Herb. Med) students at Western Sydney University a few years ago. They came as a group of nine people. They enrolled at the university because they wanted to learn to use herbal medicine. They were nervous about how to start practising, and how to start consulting. I asked for one of them to come forward and offer to be a patient in front of everyone. The woman wanting my help said she had some very difficult issues but that maybe it wasn't fair to step forward because she was actually getting help from a naturopath. I asked her to step forward and we consulted. I asked the group to not interrupt—just to make notes.

She told me that her naturopath didn't want to use herbs for her because her liver was much too sensitive and she was on all sorts of supplement pills and potions. The only herb recommended was a St Mary's thistle tablet. Two years of treatment with her naturopath gave her no progress whatsoever.

The woman had digestive difficulties starting in the stomach. The group and I discussed and designed the mix together. One suggestion they came up with for the mix was Andrographis (*Andrographis paniculata*). Why? Because she needs an astringent, was their answer.

I explained that Andrographis was also an antiviral and a very cold and strong herb—for acute cases with chronic underlying symptoms. The woman needed warming herbs and stomach help to digest her meals. Gentle tonics. She had no infection. Finally, we got to what sounded like a good mix.

Two weeks later the class and I met again. The student's difficulties were over and she was feeling great—and amazed! She was happy to take the low doses of her mix for some weeks in order to make sure she was fully repaired.

So … the primary effective qualities are taste, warmth, and moisture—and these qualities have eight separate (sub) tastes, each of which have specific energetic effects on the human body.

The secondary effective qualities describe the more specific and active effects each herb has in the body—such as restoring/relaxing, stimulating/calming, nourishing/decongesting, and these active effects of each herb will work in the person's specific organs or systems.

The tertiary effective qualities are subdivisions of the secondary qualities. They also apply to the physical/substantial and energetic aspects of each herb. The first three pairs of tertiary qualities are concerned with body substance. They are astringing/softening, solidifying/dissolving, thickening/diluting. The second two pairs are more to do with movement in the body. They are raising/sinking, dispersing/stabilising.

Then there is the tropism that designates the organs, tissue, body parts, and energetic systems—such as meridians and chakras—in which a herb has an affinity, bias or resonance.

In Greek herbal medicine traditions, each herb has a definite effect on certain body systems, tissues and parts. In Oriental medicine, a remedy is said to enter certain meridians or channels.

In Ayurvedic traditions, we have other ways of understanding the energetics. All these traditions have ways of categorising the human being in front of us and their temperaments and energies of imbalance at the time of illness, alongside their constitutional character.

The medicinal actions of each herb are a complex mixture—and the more we try to define their actions in the terminology of modern pharmaceutical science the more confusing it can become. We need the research and the descriptions of modern science because it expands our knowledge and understanding of how we can use our herbs for the benefit of humanity. It helps us to have conversations with medical scientists. We need to *add* it to our inherited traditional knowledge. We also need to have teachers of herbal medicine with 20 years plus of clinical experience alongside scientific research-based teachers, and we need to constantly seek out the wisdom and knowledge of experienced clinicians.

Traditional herbalists question thoroughly and listen carefully to the individual descriptions of how the patient's body feels. This is how we sense the physical potential of which herbs are needed to restore the patient's health. Some of our herbs are cooling, some are warming, and some are diaphoretic; the last quality, for example, warms and shifts the heat trapped in the body so as to produce sweating and thus result in cooling—like Peppermint (*Mentha piperita*). Some are warming and cooling at the same time and one theory is that the body gets to choose energetically what is needed at the time—and these are the amazing all-round healers of every single body system, such as Lavender (*Lavandula angustifolia*).

When you are designing your mix you also need to take into consideration the therapeutic categories of herbs.

Since the fourth century BC, Hippocrates distinguished three types of plant medicines: restoring nutritive substances which can be used as foods—we now know them as 'mild' herbs which can be used as gentle, long-term support; remedies or medium-strength herbs; and strong herbs which have immediate and rapid effects. These broad categories have been used in Traditional Chinese medicine for the same length of time and have formed the basis for works on pharmacology and therapeutics in European and Oriental herbal medicine for over 22 centuries.

This system of classification defines the therapeutic nature of botanicals. It directly affects herb selection and usage and provides a safe framework for the user.

Mild herbs are gentle, slow-working, cumulative and often nutritive. Weeds and medicinal foods such as Alfalfa (*Medicago sativa*), Nettle (*Urtica dioica*), Hawthorn flower (*Crataegus monogyna*), Calendula (*Calendula officinalis*), Ribwort (*Plantago lanceolata*), Dandelion (*Taraxacum officinale*), Peppermint (*Mentha piperita*), Elder flowers (*Sambucus nigra*), Chamomile (*Matricaria recutita*), Sage (*Salvia officinalis*), Goldenrod (*Solidago canadensis/virgaurea*), Comfrey (*Symphytum officinale*), Mullein (*Verbascum thapsus*), Globe artichoke (*Cynara scolymus*), Rosemary (*Rosmarinus officinalis*), Motherwort (*Leonorus cardiaca*), Lavender (*Lavandula angustifolia*), Pulsatilla (*Pulsatilla vulgaris*), Vervain (*Verbena officinalis*), Hyssop (*Hyssopus officinalis*), Marshmallow (*Althaea officinalis*), Wood betony (*Betonica officinalis*), Red clover (*Trifolium pratense*), and Lemon balm (*Melissa officinalis*) are included in this category. Some of these also have medium (or 'effective') and strong effects. For example, Motherwort is a strong antispasmodic but also a mild and medium hypotensive and nerve restorative.

Mild remedies can be used daily and taken over a long period of time to gain their full healing potential. They are restorative tonics or relaxing tonics and are not stimulating or sedative like the remedies of some of the medium-strength and strong-category herbs. They are used to prevent and to cure. For the treatment of chronic and systemic deficiency conditions, they support the vital force and are essential when vitality is depleted.

Children and the elderly often need herbs from this category exclusively. Traditional longevity formulas and elixirs all consist almost entirely of herbs in this category. They are not ineffective just because they are classified as mild. These herbs in your mixes create the fundamental physiological changes for your patients. They restore the Yin— the structure and essence, harmony and strength of the individual. Small doses of the fresh plant tinctures in this group are best.

Medium-strength herbs have both structural (Yin) and active (Yang) effects. Some can cause slightly negative side effects if used in too high doses or as too high a proportion for your mix. If used for too long also they can possess some chronic toxicity as they are cumulative. These medium-strength herbs either stimulate or sedate. Used for chronic and acute conditions of many kinds these remedies include Wormwood (*Artemesia absinthium*), Yarrow (*Achillea millefolium*), Rosemary (*Rosmarinus officinalis*), Rue (*Ruta graveolens*), Sage (*Salvia officinalis*), Burdock (*Arctium lappa*), Meadowsweet (*Filipendula ulmaria*), Parsley (*Petroselinum crispum*), Mugwort (*Artemisia vulgaris*), Red clover (*Trifolium pratense*), Elecampane (*Inula helenium*), Agrimony (*Agrimonia eupatoria*), Blue flag (*Iris versicolor*), Yellow dock (*Rumex crispus*), Valerian (*Valeriana officinalis*), Pulsatilla (*Pulsatilla vulgaris*), California poppy (*Eschscholzia californica*), Skullcap (*Scutellaria lateriflora*), and Vervain (*Verbena officinalis*).

Some of these herbs are best used for a maximum of four weeks and then discontinued. Or used in small amounts in the herb mix. If carefully mixed with certain mild herbs the cumulative toxicity can be entirely avoided.

Strong herbs have very active or Yang effects that are rapid. Some can cause immediate side effects and negative reactions (known to some as a cleansing reaction), and some can possess acute toxicity when used alone in doses that are too high for the individual. These remedies cause powerful stimulation or sedation and are most often used for the treatment of symptoms rather than causes. Therapeutically they are draining and used for the symptom treatment of severe advanced conditions.

Appropriate also for severe acute conditions, they can deal directly and immediately with pathogenic elements. They should only be used with care and in very small doses mixed with other mild herbs to support the body and when the possible side effects are understood.

For example, I don't believe Goldenseal should ever be used alone. The side effects are much too painful in the wrong dose for the individual and have been dramatic for me personally. Poke root is another dramatic, strong herb.

If I am using a strong herb for a patient, I mix carefully in low amounts in my mixes with 11 herbs in, and I would use plenty of carefully chosen mild herbs that support the body at the same time so as not to risk overwhelming the patient.

I was never taught these philosophies. I learned them myself through experiencing the direct effect of Traditional Chinese herbal medicine on my body during some serious illnesses and through the kindness of the herbalists treating me in Chinatown, Sydney. They were good enough to answer my endless questions as I watched the dried herbs for my prescription being measured out and popped in the paper packages assigned for each day's dose.

I also learned through working for many years alongside a wonderful Chinese herbalist and acupuncturist in the Blue Mountains. He was my personal therapist and we shared clinic rooms in Katoomba. He and his wife are still close friends and he shares his knowledge and his Chinese Materia Medica books in English with me.

I also learned these philosophies by reading over and over the wonderful two-volume book by Peter Holmes, *The Energetics of Western Herbal Medicine*. These books have given me a familiarity with how a human being functions on all levels—structurally, physiologically, emotionally—and how an under-functioning organ or system can be responsible for creating moods and sometimes deep emotional turmoil or depression. I consider this knowledge gathered together from traditional clinical practice of Eastern and Western Herbal Medicine vital to be an effective herbalist.

Matthew Wood has written wonderful things to share about the herbal philosophies from our history—and about the magic, alchemy and mystery of our history. He writes for us about the character of the herbs and which systems and organs they like to help us with.

Dorothy Hall writes for us about the characters of our patients and how important the energetics of the cosmos are in our work. She teaches us how sun sign astrology can help us understand the vitality of our patients and how life's challenges might affect them; that knowing current planetary transits can help us understand, question and diagnose any emotional causes of illness in our patients.

Sajah Popham has written *Evolutionary Herbalism* which is restoring some of our authentic history and our spiritual connection to the Earth and plant medicine. He also explains our philosophies. I can't read it—it's too academic for me. I love that some of my students are enthusiastically getting support for their work with herbs from it, though.

I learned much from Glyn Braddy at the International Academy of Alchemists in the 1980s—he taught me so many mysterious, energetic, shamanic, and unscientific things that I use in my work, including Kinesiology.

For those of you who have been trained to take a calculator and their anxiety into the mixing and dispensing area of your clinic, please see the following mathematical logic. It should appease your anxiety and help you open your hearts and allow your intuition to come through. Awakening your intuition will enhance your ability to connect meaningfully with your patient—and this will assist you in making the very best mix for them.

I want to demonstrate that if any of you have been taught to use more than 5 ml doses, with only five herbs in a 200 ml bottle you could be regularly using more than the *British Herbal Pharmacopoeia* (*BHP*) recommended safe doses.

Let us assume that 25–30 drops is approximately 1 ml, keeping in mind this is not precise, as the size of the drops differs depending on the viscosity of each herb tincture.

Because each 200 ml bottle actually holds 220 ml, the herb mix is made up of 44 ml of each of the five herbs.

Using the dosage of 30 drops three times daily The patient is therefore taking 90 drops daily = 3.5 ml daily

The patient is having 6 drops of each of the five herbs in each dose which is 18 drops of each herb daily. This is not even 1 ml of each of the herbs daily. This low dose (considered non-therapeutic by some) is well within the safety recommendations of the *BHP* for almost any herb.

Example 1: To treat a patient with long-term chronic illness

First, we want to give them a lift and then a long, gentle, building of strength and repair.

We take a 220 ml mix with 44 ml of each of the five herbs.

The dosage is 40 drops five times daily for two weeks then drop back to three times daily.

Now the patient is taking 200 drops daily = 8 ml daily for two weeks. They are having 40 drops of each herb daily = 1.5 ml of each herb daily.

More than likely this is still within the guidelines of the *BHP* recommended doses of each herb for *safety*.

Example 2: To treat a patient with an acute illness

We make a 220 ml mix with 44 ml of each of five herbs.

At a dosage of 40 drops every hour for a max of ten doses daily our patient is taking 8 drops of each herb every hour. And 400 drops daily = 16 ml daily.

So the patient is having 80 drops of each herb daily = 3.3 ml of each herb daily.

This could be too high according to the BHP dosage for safety recommendations.

Using my method

Mixing 11 herbs in a 220 ml bottle (a 200 ml bottle actually has space for 220 ml).

My 220 ml mixes are mostly made with 20 ml of each of 11 herbs.

The dosage is 2–3 ml (60–90 drops) three times daily.

The patient is taking 180–270 drops daily = 6–9 ml daily.

My patient is having 16–24 drops of each herb daily = not even 1 ml of each herb daily. This is well within safe dose recommendations for each herb, whether they are mild, medium or strong herbs.

CHAPTER TWENTY ONE

The importance of manufacturing processes

In my practice I have found the effectiveness of my herbal mixes depends first on the quality of my medicines. Back in 1985 the Nature Spirit 1:8 tinctures seemed to work fine.

The herbal material used to make these tinctures was mostly imported from Europe and in 1986 the Chernobyl nuclear disaster happened and our herbal imports were found by customs to be radioactive. Now we had to find new sources of herbal plant material and a new awareness developed around where our plants came from. Having to provide our own medicinal herbs as much as possible helped our Australian herbal farming industry to begin.

In 1988 Australia got two new manufacturing companies—the Herbal Extract Company founded by Lyndsay Shume, a fourth-generation herbalist, and Green Pharm, both using the traditional manufacturing system of maceration. Green Pharm tinctures were made with plants harvested from a cooperative of organic growers in Victoria. They were dried fast and made into tinctures on the property.

Greg Whitten was the inspiration behind the growing and manufacturing and he helped them create a cooperative of organic herb growers. We know them today as Southern Light Herbs. Natalie and Michael head up the cooperative these days and teach workshops on the organic growing of medicinal herbs. They now have 20 certified organic farms all over Australia producing the herbs for tea mixes and selling them to herbalists for medicine making.

Greg bought a farm in Tasmania to grow his herbs and slowly became the maker of tinctures for Gould's pharmacy in Hobart. Greg is one of our much respected elders here in Australia and his book, *Herbal Harvest*, is the most comprehensive book available, in the English language, on organic herb production for the manufacture of herbal medicines.

Changing from the use of Nature Spirit tinctures to these rich and powerful blends from the Herbal Extract Company with their 1:1 tinctures, and Green Pharm who made tinctures of 1:1, 1:2, and 1:5, and a few succi (plural of succus), juices made from the fresh plant, was such a joy.

I was given helpful advice from Michael and Linda Gardiner at Green Pharm. When I asked Michael for advice on dosing, he said, 'Well if you use five 1:8 tinctures in your 100 ml mix, and dose recommendations of 25–30 drops (which equals 1 ml), why can't you use ten 1:1, 1:2, or 1:3 tinctures in a mix and 30–60 drop doses (which equals 1–2 ml)?'

This worked for me and meant that I could expand my creative thoughts about how many tinctures I could mix together for each patient. It made better sense to me and seemed to be more aligned with the Chinese ideas of *Go easy, go gentle, and stay in tune with the patterns of presenting symptoms of the individual*. This also aligned with Dorothy Hall teaching us to avoid pushing the patient's body out of balance in a new way by dosing too high.

Suddenly I had available to me herbal medicines made with the traditional method of maceration for some months from the Herbal Extract Company, and Green Pharm with their organic plants grown in Australia and made into tinctures on the farm. My patients had wonderful reports of easy shifts in their ailments. And my dosing began to increase a little. I found the lives of my patients were often so busy that all they could manage to take were two doses daily. I increased my doses to 1–2 ml twice a day of a mix with 11 herbs. I got wonderful results—gentle and fast.

Once I had moved to Blue Mountains in 1992, I became known as the village herbalist (as I described in Chapter 1) and I started making my own medicines from my happy, organically grown, fresh herbs in my cottage garden. Michael and Linda Gardner kindly guided me by telephone on how to make my herbal tinctures. I made them with fresh

THE IMPORTANCE OF MANUFACTURING PROCESSES   125

plants straight from my garden and I began using them on my patients. I used my plants straight from the Earth. I felt that the vital force was still alive and that the plant water still held inside the plant was an important part of their healing force.

Manufacturers of herbal medicines on a large scale can't really do this. They are handling massive amounts of plant material. The risk of mould growing and bacteria flourishing in the plants awaiting maceration is too great. This is one reason why plants are harvested on farms and dried fast on large mesh trays in massive rooms with low heating and fans. This speeds up the drying and keeps the air moving.

The aim is to have the material dry in two to four days. When it is tested to be beyond risk of any dampness it will be packaged in airtight containers and shipped as fast as possible to the manufacturers of the tinctures. There it will be opened and examined, and samples from different sections of the package will then be sent to the laboratory to be checked. If any damp is found, or bacteria or mould is discovered, the plant material will be rejected.

I got busier and busier and my clients from Sydney drove up to the Blue Mountains for their consultations. The reports of better results with fresh plant medicines just kept coming. And my dosing knowledge expanded. Still, I was regularly using 30 drops two to six times a day depending on the condition, the patient and their vital force, and what I wanted the mix to do. I began seeing many people in their 80s and this made me a bit nervous in case they were frail. Sometimes I prescribe 2–3ml doses two to four times a day. My favourite amount of herbs in my mixes began to consistently be 11. I believe it's my magic number.

After 18 years of running a busy clinical practice, I began to teach herbal medicine at Nature Care College in Sydney and the Australasian College of Natural Therapies (ACNT), and then I went to Coffs Harbour to teach at the NSW College of Natural Medicine. At the same time, I kept my practice going. My practice has been the seat of my learning and the source of loving nourishment in my world. Being needed and appreciated feeds my heart.

In Australia now (2024) we have medicinal tinctures made from dried plants and manufactured by percolation which is a more modern method of production created by pharmacy. Production is faster and doesn't favour saturation or the use of fresh plant material. I like maceration myself and it's the method I use to manufacture my tinctures with fresh plants which I have either grown myself or wildcrafted from places with clean earth.

However, there are now also a number of manufacturing companies in Australia that use the traditional manufacturing process of maceration of plant material in a solvent mix for a number of weeks. This means the herbs are really soaking up the solvent and the plant cells are being saturated over and over again, which makes them explode more of their ingredients out into the liquid.

The companies that use the traditional method of maceration—the Herbal Extract Company, Pharmaceutical Plant Company (PPC), and Optimal Rx—involve themselves in supporting organic farmers in Australia and around the world by purchasing their herbal material to make their tinctures for us. They are very fussy about checking the quality of the dried herbs that arrive for them to use—how well they have been dried and what properties are still alive in the plant material.

One of these companies, PPC supports and distributes the medicine made on an organically certified farm, Marleen Herbs of Tasmania. The European family who created the farm came from a long history of organic farming and making herbal medicines for the European market. Making the tinctures on-site with the traditional methods described above allows them to use the plants just harvested on the farm.

Our Australian organic growers work hard to bring us high-quality herbs dried fast and efficiently, and the quality control at the manufacturing centre/laboratory is very thorough. You can visit these manufacturers and be shown around their production facilities. You can also visit the farms.

In my experience and with the feedback from my patients over the years, I feel sure that the dosage we recommend depends first on the manufacturing methods of your medicines, whether the plant material used is fresh or dried, and how long it has been dried for. It is worth repeating this point.

That they all work—fresh or dried, macerated or percolated, boiled or cold percolated, in infusions and decoctions, and in tinctures made with alcohol or apple cider vinegar—is an incredible tribute to the power and the magic of the plants themselves. Of course, the creation of the herbal mix for the individual patient by a skilful prescribing herbalist/magician/alchemist is also vitally important.

CHAPTER TWENTY TWO

Who tells you what doses to use?

In the history and traditions of herbal medicine, stretching back thousands of years, the skills of mixing and dosing were learned over many years during an apprenticeship to a skilled and successful clinician. An apprenticeship was gained by working for the busy herbalist, or medicine woman, and closely assisting them in their work of making medicines and healing people with these medicines. Historically, in all cultures, a herbalist-to-be was taught only by an experienced herbalist while working directly with patients.

In turn, the experienced herbalist had studied with a master and then developed their knowledge and skills from working closely with individual patients over many years—regularly questioning the patient about the effects of mixes and simples (one single herb) and keeping precise notes from these answers and observations, as well as storing these details in their heart and in the memory of their senses.

Of course, the writing down part of this ideal picture only happened if the medicine woman or man could write—which wasn't a common skill in olden times. And the Celts believed this knowledge shouldn't be written down because it would be stolen from them and used wrongly. They believed their knowledge made them valued by their tribe and cared for by their community.

The herbalists, or medicine men and women, watched and listened carefully to each patient describing the feelings and functions of their body, and then to the changes taking place with each dose of herbal medicine. This close relationship between the herbalist and the patient is how the growth of this knowledge happens. Thus the inherited knowledge is built on, described and handed down to the apprentice, who then adds to it while using it for their own herbal/healing practice. This apprenticeship needs to take around ten years.

The master teacher cannot let them loose on their community until they are seen to be ready. Otherwise both the teacher and student will lose their status in the community and the trust their people have for them. Respect for their teacher was inbuilt because their reputation came from who taught them. So acknowledgement of their teacher was natural and inherited. This knowledge that is handed down from teacher to apprentice is our inherited body of information—how the plants affect the human body. This is the traditional knowledge that tells us how to use the herbs in clinical practice and the subtle differences in how each body uses the herbs to repair.

All this development and growth of knowledge has been written down by great herbal doctors of history: Galen (129–216 AD), Avicenna (Ibn Sina) (980–1037 AD) in Persia, known as the Father of Early Modern Medicine), Hildegard of Bingen (1098–1179), Trota of Salerno (the world's first gynaecologist living in the early or middle decades of the twelfth century), Paracelsus (1493–1541), and Nicholas Culpeper (1616–1654). All of these people were from wealthy families with the advantage of having learned how to write.

Way back before BC became AD, the social status of the healers was akin to the status of priests, walking side by side with the tribal leaders. In some cultures, the healers were also the spiritual leaders/priests.

Slowly, slowly, the invasion of the Christian church and the insidious influence of their takeover of the souls, religions, and social systems—and lands of the wealthy—reduced the status of the healers to 'evil pagans' working against God's intention for you: if you had sickness, God had sent it to you. This belief grew until it became the excuse for burning and hanging the healers of Europe and further afield, as well as confiscating their lands and destroying any writings they may have had. This went on for about 400 years.

The long and complicated history and development of European Herbal Medicine begins with the Egyptians and the Celts around 1500 BC (as far as we have written evidence). This history and the precision of the descriptions of what results the herbs had on the human body actually underpins the growth and development of pharmacy, surgery, homoeopathy, modern medicine, theosophical medicine, and flower essence therapy and is beyond the scope of this book.

In traditional herbal medicine we are still using hundreds of herbs for the same symptoms as described by the Egyptians in the writings found in the Temple of Isis.

As a clinician, my work here is to add my knowledge, observations, and studies to our body of work in order to support the use and growth of the Empirical Science of Traditional Herbal Medicine. Each country and each culture developed their herbal traditions. I acknowledge the elders and custodians of this knowledge in all cultures. In my work, I like to acknowledge my teachers and my focus is on European traditions as this is my heritage.

In more modern times some of our great practising traditional herbalists have written for us from their clinical experience—Maurice Messegué, Juliette de Baïracli Levy, Dorothy Hall, Michael Tierra, David Hoffmann, Farida Sharan, Susun Weed, Peter Holmes, Matthew Wood and Paul Bergner, amongst others, have all added their knowledge to the old knowledge. Their writings are summaries and details from their own healing stories and clinical work while using the old knowledge as a baseline. All of them give us unique and important information, founded on practical experience; and some give us their case studies as well.

Hardly any of these writers tell you much about creative and effective dosing in their writings. Why? Because it depends on the herbs used in the mix (synergy) and the pattern of symptoms to be treated. This art can only be learned from a clinician *while* treating the patterns of the illness and the conditions of each individual patient. And because the mixes and doses needed daily for an acute illness can change hourly. It's complicated.

So how do we learn the skills of mixing and dosing today? Since 2003 I have been teaching herbal therapeutics, manufacturing, and clinical practice to herbal medicine students as well as mentoring them. In this time I have come across many people employed to teach herbal medicine with no questions asked about how many years of clinical practice experience they have had. Neither has there been any requirement that while teaching they must maintain their clinical practice. Over the years I have met many teachers of herbal medicine who began teaching before they had finished studying or in the first year after finishing their studies. This is not good enough.

Many of these people with no clinical experience have been involved in deciding how we should be teaching herbal medicine in our colleges and universities today! Self-appointed authorities, they decide what we should teach about the herbs and which herbs should stay in our repertoire and which herbs should be thrown out. Some of these people have also been advising and helping to create our manufacturing companies.

This has left me with many questions about what our naturopaths and herbalists have been taught, and by whom, and who is benefiting. Here are some of my questions:

- *How do our students learn about mixing and dosing?*
- *Who is teaching them about mixing and dosing and how did the teacher know?*
- *Why don't we learn to dose by the conditions and symptomology of the body?*
- *Why don't we learn to mix for different conditions and different body types?*
- *Why don't we learn to dose for acute and chronic conditions differently?*
- *What happened to our traditional focus on individuals?*
- *What has happened to the philosophies of vitalism and energetic disharmony?*
- *Why have mixing and dosing been reduced to a simplistic chart with daily or weekly doses to be worked out with a calculator? Where did this information come from?*

CHAPTER TWENTY THREE

The influence of the *British Herbal Pharmacopoeia*

First, let's think about why you are given dosing recommendations—or are they restrictions?—the ones on your herbal medicine bottles and the ones on your charts. Why were they developed and when?

In the late 1970s and early 1980s, governments in England and Australia began trying to legislate against herbal medicine and naturopathy, trying to stop herbalists from practising and health shops selling. There was such a public outcry, and this led to the formation of committees to examine the products for the protection of the public.

If you look at the Preface in the 1983 edition of the *British Herbal Pharmacopoeia* you will see the names of the committee that put together the pharmacopoeia, along with their qualifications.

Mostly they are pharmacists and scientists. Two of the nine are members of the National Institute of Medical Herbalists (NIMH). Fletcher-Hyde is fascinating—Google him and see. He was the son of a herbalist in Leicester and a chemistry and botany graduate of 1932. He was Director of Research at the National Institute of Herbal Medicine for more than 30 years and held a doctorate in Botanical Medicine from the London School of Botanical Medicine.

In the 1930s students of pharmacy were trained to use herbal medicine. They would make up mixes for the conditions described by a doctor in a letter given to the patient to take to their local pharmacist. This was like a prescription but pharmaceutical companies didn't make many standardised drugs then. So pharmacists and doctors used herbal medicine in their treatments.

In 1964 the British Herbal Medicine Association (BHMA) was founded 'to advance the science and practice of herbal medicine in the UK'. MPS is the Medical Protection Society.

In 1968 the Medicines Act was passed in the UK and the world of herbal medicine was challenged. Could it be considered therapeutic or indeed even medicinal? The BHMA managed to keep herbal medicine on the therapeutic medicines list in the Act.

Then the world of Fletcher-Hyde and other botanical medicine practitioners, including chemists, the BHMA, and many other scientists, came together and created the *British Herbal Pharmacopoeia*. It took them years of hard work to collect evidence and information. Their first edition came out in 1983. They kept gathering information and produced a second edition in 1990.

General references cited are from *Martindale*, which describes the properties of plants and their extracts; and Jackson and Snowdon's *Atlas of Microscopy of Medicinal Plants, Culinary Herbs and Spices*, which is a botany and manufacturing textbook. These are both pharmacists' textbooks for manufacturing medicines.

The *British Herbal Pharmacopoeia* was created as a guidebook for safety compiled by an advisory committee of scientists, botanists, doctors, and pharmacists with some help from the National Institute of Medical Herbalists. It was *not* compiled by a group of herbalists based on clinical practice. Two members of the committee were herbalists with empirical knowledge and clinical experience; they were not appointed to work out effective dosing—only safety. The committee compiled this reference book to begin protecting the public and to make manufacturers and practitioners liable for public safety.

The BHMA describes itself as:

> *The UK representative of the European Scientific Cooperative on Phytotherapy (ESCOP), the body that has become recognised by the European Medicines Agency as providing the leading scientific resources on the therapeutic use of herbal medicinal products in the European Union.*

> *Members of the BHMA include companies involved in the manufacture or supply of herbal medicines, herbal practitioners, academics, pharmacists, students of phytotherapy, and others. The BHMA has supported these members with advice and comments on legislation and labelling from the beginning.*

So when the Australian Therapeutic Goods Administration (TGA) came into being they too were concerned with how to make manufacturers responsible for the safety of the public so they required expiry dates and that the dosage ranges should be on the bottles—and these dosage ranges were taken from the *BHP*. Following advice from scientists concerned to keep the public safe. Otherwise, where would it come from?

We all know that expiry dates are a stab in the dark. The medicines are almost all 50 per cent ethanol alcohol or more—they will take many years to go off or stop being effective. Before 1990 we had no expiry dates on our medicines.

Now we have dosage charts based on the *BHP* recommendations, handed out with warnings in college by teachers who may not have used herbal medicines in a clinical setting at all. Some of them have science degrees and no clinical experience.

So who *would* be experienced enough to teach you the skills of effective dosing?

A practising herbalist with at least 20 years of clinical experience is really your obvious answer. A student would ideally be an apprentice to a herbalist or teacher with a busy clinic, as in the old days. A ten-year apprenticeship should do it!

To use these charted dosage ranges for your prescribing guidelines is too restrictive for a practitioner. Look at Valerian (*Valeriana officinalis*) or Lavender (*Lavandula angustifolia*)—you have to consider what you are using it for to work out what doses you might use.

At the Sydney 1995 NHAA International Conference in a talk given by Hein Zeylstra, he told us a story from his clinical practice that demonstrates my point. He found a woman in his waiting room very flustered and, knowing her case involved high blood pressure (BP), he told her he needed to take her BP and that she had at least one hour to wait for her appointment. Her BP was far too high so he mixed up a drink of water for her with 75 ml Valerian and 75 ml Crampbark (*Viburnum opulus*). After telling her to sip it slowly, he left her there waiting.

When he came back an hour later her BP had hardly shifted. He repeated the drink with the same amounts of Valerian and Crampbark and told her she had to wait another hour while she sipped it slowly. Back he came an hour later and checked her BP again. It had decreased slightly.

He repeated the drink for a third time and left her for another hour. When he came back three hours had passed in total, and three drinks. This equalled 450 ml of the herb mix (225 ml each of Valerian and Crampbark) in one afternoon. Now her BP was down to normal. Amazing that she was awake and could still walk!

However, the *BHP* says to give 0.3–1 ml three times daily of a 1:1 Valerian tincture, and doesn't tell us if this is fresh plant tincture or dried. The dose of Crampbark recommended by the *BHP* is 2–4 ml three times daily of a 1:1 tincture.

Hein Zeylstra was born in 1929 in Amsterdam and became involved with the growing of medicinal herbs. He subsequently studied herbal medicine at NIMH in the UK and in 1977 he founded the School of Herbal Medicine which later became the College of Phytotherapy. He ran a busy clinic for more than 20 years and taught many of the well-known herbalists of today who now live and work in the US, Canada, Ireland, New Zealand, and Australia.

Do you think Hein Zeylstra damaged his client with these doses? Or do you think he used the herbs with the experience of a traditional herbal medicine practitioner and the full knowledge of what this patient needed? With these particular herbs, the hypertensive patient would have been a bit sleepy and floppy by the time she got to her consultation!

I used this story years later to try and bring my own BP down. My reading at the time was 215/105. I couldn't face drinking the tincture with that amount of ethanol alcohol so I used 2,000 mg tablets of Valerian. I took one tablet every half hour. It took some hours but after five hours and ten of these tablets, my BP monitor finally gave me a reading of normal.

In my clinical practice, I have found the following: if you are giving a nervous client help to sit an exam, you might give them 5 ml of Lavender and Rosemary combined every hour for a few hours before the exam. This is not the dose recommended by the *BHP*.

A sleep mix for a patient has to contain the best mix of herbs for that patient. There are many nervines and each of them works in the nervous system along different pathways and you may need to prescribe as little as 30 drops every hour after dinner and before bed—or 5 ml three times after dinner and before bed. Or you may need to start this patient taking their doses before dinner. So much depends on your patient and what their lifestyle and the stresses in their lives are. They may need a mix of well-chosen nervines, along with other herbs, to take all day to assist them in winding down slowly, depending on how many years they have been feeling under stress.

And then there are pain relief mixes and so on. A pain relief mix to take before going to the dentist I would make with approximately five pain relief herbs. If, like me, you can't cope with the steroid-based anti-pain injections, I would recommend you take 5 ml doses every half hour for two or three hours, making sure someone else is driving you to the dentist and bringing you home.

Now that herbalists are being educated to use dosage charts—which to me is a silly and distracting idea—manufacturers are expected, even obliged, to provide these. You are being taught that the recommended doses on your chart show you the lowest dose required for efficiency and the maximum dose for safety. This seems to be how the chart is understood. I would consider this a massive misunderstanding seemingly perpetuated by teachers who have little, if any, clinical experience.

Back to the *BHP*. The research used to compile this manual for the protection of the public was not based on studying the effects of whole plants on human bodies—it was based on pharmacy and was useful for manufacturers, botanists and pharmacists. The amount of data for herbalists in this book is extremely limited. Have a look at the information. As a practitioner, is it helpful?

Then have a look at a herbal therapeutics book based on traditional information about how a plant will affect the human body. Peter Holmes has written for us the most thoroughly researched and referenced work we have available to us for our clinical practice. *The Energetics of Western Herbal Medicine* has the most brilliant information on dosing I have found. Then there is your patient. Many of them will be able to tell you in detail how their body is changing in response to the herbal medicine.

Do I use dosing charts? Never. My starting-out ability to prescribe, mix, and dose came directly from my teachers, their traditional information and their clinical experience. My knowledge has developed through listening to my patients, asking precise questions, referring to books written by experienced traditional herbalists, and through my direct experience of working with my patients and myself with herbal medicines.

CHAPTER TWENTY FOUR

Case studies

Case 1: A tropical infection

Early in my professional life, I was asked to treat someone with a serious tropical infection caught in the jungles of South America while filming a documentary. I did know her, but not well. She came from one of Australia's wealthy influential families. She had been in and out of hospital for six months and was desperate. The trips to the hospital left her without effective help because the doctors couldn't identify the pathogen. So they didn't know what to treat her with. They sent her home and told her there was no point in coming back. She was so sick she believed she was going to die.

Her raging fevers got worse and became more and more dangerous to her, damaging her life force in a wild attempt to beat the infection in a body already totally exhausted; the infection was spreading and damaging her internal organs and systems. How could I turn her away? She had nowhere to turn for help. After putting her in my spare room bed I watched and responded to her fevers and body condition about every half hour for three days—in the night as well as the daytime.

Using three different mixes I gave her 30 drops from each of the three mixes every half hour, depending on her state at the time. The terrible waves of sweating heat and the intensely shivering, freezing cold happened at the same time with awful shaking that left her body wasted. These episodes lasted seven to ten minutes and were happening every ten minutes when she arrived at my door. It took me a few hours to get them to calm down and become further apart. After about 12 hours they were less intense, less worrying and much further apart.

However, a big crisis occurred on the second night and she got worse again. I could only keep doing my best with herbs every 30 minutes to one hour. I don't often pray but I did on this night. She was still with me in the morning and by the third night her fevers had diminished to really far apart and not very intense. That second night with her was frightening; I thought this was the end of my career as a herbalist. This woman went home better on the fifth day and never relapsed into those awful fevers. She was amazed, very grateful and kept in touch for some years.

This was the end of my nervousness about the power of herbs and the beginning of my courageous conviction to always try to help but never to claim loudly that I knew what I was doing or that I could treat a medically named illness. And the beginning of my realisation that to talk about 30-drop doses as 'not therapeutic' or as 'ineffective' is totally ridiculous.

If I counted up the amount of millilitres I had given the woman with the tropical infection in one 12-hour period it would have added up to a large amount. But my mixes contained many different herbs and, although I may have exceeded the *BHP* daily recommended dose of some of the herbs, I watched carefully for the patient's response and gave very small doses each time. No one could derisively call me a drop-dose herbalist!

Case 2: A deep cyst

In the first year of my clinical practice, a woman came for a morning consultation and said that a large and deep cyst had been slowly forming behind her ear. Separate from her Main Mix of herbal repair, I made her a 50 ml mix of Horsetail (*Equisetum arvense*), Poke root (*Phytolacca* spp.), and Fenugreek (*Trigonella foenum-graecum*)—equal amounts— and told her to take 10 drops in a little water every hour on an empty stomach. The next day she called me. She had taken this dose all day— seven times before bed. She woke at 3 am with the terrible smell of the burst cyst all over her pillow.

Case 3: Pelvic inflammatory infection

Recently one of my mentees, a fine naturopath herself, emailed me about what she thought was a pelvic inflammatory infection pain. Her email said:

> So just this last 3–4 days I have had left lower abdomen tenderness and mild pain. At first, I thought it was because I had eaten way too many seed crackers and they had gotten stuck in my guts! But somehow I don't think this is the issue now. My bowels have been normal and I have been going 2–3 times a day which is normal for me.
>
> So I am starting to think it's pelvic infection again as it seems to be following the same pattern as last time. I don't have any other symptoms yet but feeling a bit tired. I think if it is the pelvic infection coming back again I will start getting unwell over the next few days. I don't really want to go to the doctor because I'm so over the internal ultrasounds etc. and antibiotics, so I think I would be wise to treat this as a pelvic infection.

On the same day, I answered:

> I do remember our conversation at the workshop early this year and am really happy to have a talk about it this afternoon—after about 1:30 pm I'm free. Any good? Meanwhile, I can recommend you getting stuck into this mix of herbs: 110 ml—Horsetail 20 ml, Poke root 10 ml, Calendula 15 ml, Plantain 20 ml, Echinacea (Echinacea spp.) 25 ml, Red clover 20 ml.
> Dose: 15 drops every hour.
> I'm available in the morning tomorrow as well. Let me know?

She texted that she didn't need to talk to me the next day. In another text three days later she was doing fine. She sent this email with her thanks:

> So just checking in to let you know how I'm going—I'm feeling wonderful now! The tenderness seems to have completely gone. It was either late Friday or Saturday I felt a funny sensation in the sore area, kind of like something was stuck together and suddenly 'unstuck' or maybe popped. So I'm wondering if I had an ovarian cyst. Anyway, you're amazing and I feel great. Do you think I should continue on the mix as a preventative for now to be sure it's all cleared up?

My answer was:

> Yes. Could have been an ovarian cyst, could have been a blocked lymph gland in the groin area that became infected. Let's just get your lower body cleaned out through the lymph system. Just reduce the dose to 15 drops twice a day. Take until the mix is finished.

To mix for the individual and to recommend doses that are effective, we need to ask a lot of questions and listen to patients and think about the patterns of their symptoms. We need to reconnect with the energetics of the herbs and their traditional uses, and the patterns of symptoms that the herbs work in. Otherwise, how do we choose which bronchial decongestant herb is the best one to use for the individual in front of us? How do we choose which liver-restoring herb is best?

Case 4: Toxic overload, Candida, diabetes, joint, and digestive issues

On 20 August 2001, BT, aged 57, came to see me with no hair, toxic overload, painful joints, digestive difficulties, and diabetes after a four-month stay in hospital for a 'standard hysterectomy'.

A strong, positive, and vital woman, BT was a full-time working grandmother with a large, healthy family. She was a caring and respected member of the community in the upper Blue Mountains. I had known her for ten years and she sent me patients but hardly ever needed my herbalist support herself.

BT went to the hospital for a hysterectomy after three months of heavy, non-stop bleeding that had seemed unresponsive to the herbal medicine I made for her. After the surgery a serious infection set in and she spent four months in hospital, with drainage tubes needed to clean out the peritonitis.

For four months she was given antibiotics by mouth and intravenously. Flagyl was used for weeks at a time even though it caused her diarrhoea and vomiting. BT came out of hospital with diabetes, high BP, and medication for both; she also had extreme digestive problems with severe fungal growth on her mouth and tongue, vagina and anus. Most of her hair had fallen out and she had lost a substantial amount of weight and muscle tone. She looked pregnant and was very uncomfortable and swollen in the belly.

She had been taking Zyloprim to prevent kidney stones and arthritic joints from her late 30s until now—some 27 years. In the Australian MIMS, they explain that Zyloprim should not be taken with high BP or when liver damage exists; when I explained this, BT stopped taking it. She also was not happy to be on pharmaceuticals for high BP and diabetes. I told her to be careful with this and to make sure she had the supervision of an agreeable and supportive doctor when she felt ready to come off these medications.

Anti-Candida Herb Mix – 100 ml

To clean up the Candida overgrowth and gently begin supporting her recovery. Also to help with detoxing, immune restoration and liver repair.

Pau d'arco 15 ml, Calendula 15 ml, Peppermint 10 ml, Poke root 5 ml, Goldenseal 10 ml, Gymnema 15 ml, Fennel 15 ml, Figwort 15 ml.

Dose: 2 ml (50 drops) three times a day, 20 minutes before meals.

Supplements: EPA/DHA – one capsule three times a day with a meal.

HaemoRed – one with each meal.

Tresos B – one tablet twice a day with breakfast and lunch.

Magoro – one tablet twice a day with breakfast and lunch.

Activgestion – one with each meal.

Diet: No wheat, no dairy, and easy food combined as in *Fit for Life*. Animal protein in every meal—goat's and sheep's cheeses and yoghurts, eggs count too. For snacks—nuts. Only whole grains, vary the grains you eat.

My reasons for using some of the herbs I gave BT

20 August 2001

Mix 1 – 110 ml

This mix I gave her for cleaning out the fungal/Candida overgrowth, clearing the inevitable lymph congestion, drying up the dampness through her digestive system so it could start working again, restoring her liver to clean the blood, and starting to rebuild her system.

Pau d'arco – mild herb, bitter and cold, stimulates, restores, astringes, and decongests in the intestines, lungs, veins, kidney, bladder, and blood. The antidote to poisons as well as antibacterial, antifungal, antiviral, and antiparasitic.

Calendula – mild herb, a bit bitter, sweet, salty, and pungent, neutral with cooling potential, dry, decongesting, astringing, stimulating, softening, and dissolving in the liver, heart, uterus, skin, veins, lymph, and blood. Increases oestrogen and is good for post-menopause. Also antibacterial, and antifungal.

Peppermint – mild- to medium-strength herb, pungent, a bit sweet, warm with secondary cooling effect, dry, stimulating, dispersing, restoring, astringing, relaxing in the head, heart, lungs, stomach, intestines, gall bladder, liver, uterus, nerves. This is a minor percentage of the mix.

Poke root – strong herb with some chronic toxicity, a bit pungent and sweet, neutral, softening, dissolving and stimulating in the digestive, lymphatic and musculoskeletal systems. This is a very small percentage of the mix and the action is supported by mild herbs.

Goldenseal – strong herb with some chronic toxicity, bitter and astringent, cold, dry, decongesting, astringing, stabilising, restoring, stimulating in the stomach, intestines, lungs, heart, reproductive organs, bladder, kidneys, liver, gallbladder. This is a very small percentage of the mix and the action is supported by medium-strength herbs.

Fennel – mild herb, a bit pungent and sweet, warm and dry, tonic for relaxing, restoring, astringing bladder, spleen, stomach, intestines, and lungs. For appetite loss.

Gymnema – mild herb used to reduce blood sugar after meals and eliminate sugar cravings. It is believed to stimulate insulin production in the pancreas and promote regeneration of insulin-producing islet cells.

Figwort – mild herb, bitter, a bit pungent, cool and dry, dissolving and decongesting for the liver, kidneys, intestines, pancreas, blood and lymph. For oedema, constipation, pancreas insufficiency, and diabetes.

3 September 2001

Diabetes readings improved lots and feeling great. Got energy and colour. Hair still falling out. Tongue very improved.

Repeated everything. Added Cytobifidus three times a day before meals.

29 September 2001

Going real good. Hair still falling out. Seems like time to change the herb mix but keep supporting her system to continue the Candida and fungus clean-up, along with organ repair. Here we can increase the doses a little because of the added tonics.

Anti-Candida, Antifungal, Antibacterial, Gut Repair Mix 2 – 220 ml

Nettle 20 ml, Horsetail 20 ml, Parsley 20 ml, Pau d'arco (*Tabebuia impetiginosa*) 20 ml, Calendula 20 ml, Rosemary 20 ml, Poke root 10 ml, Goldenseal 10 ml, Figwort (*Scrophularia nodosa*) 20 ml, Fennel (*Foeniculum vulgare*) 20 ml, Gymnema 20 ml, Globe artichoke 20 ml.

Dose: 3 ml twice a day.

Supplements: Tresos B – one a day with breakfast, EPA/DHA – one with breakfast.

Ultra Muscleze – 1 teaspoon three times a week.

100 ml mix of Rosemary oil 40ml with Hypericum oil 60 ml. Massage head daily.

8 February 2002

No more diabetes or blood pressure medication needed. Feeling great. Hair growth happening.

Repeat last mix – Dandelion root instead of Fennel. Same supplements.

BT also started taking her partner's herbal bronchitis mix a couple of times a week to prevent respiratory infections.

She believed that six months of rubbing the Rosemary oil into her head was restoring her hair growth. I believed it was because the internal herbal mix was restoring her body from the awful damage done by the treatment she ended up needing in hospital.

I like to imagine that if BT had been treated concurrently by an experienced herbalist with herbal medicine while in hospital she would not have sustained such incredible damage and would have been out of hospital in just a few weeks.

BT stayed on this mix until 7 December 2004 and sometimes got the Tresos B, the Ultra Muscleze and the EPA/DHA. She noted that any deviation from her diet for long, such as eating cakes, affected her blood sugar readings, so she became better and better at making good choices for comfort and health safety.

7 December 2004

BT wanted 500 ml of her herbal medicine because she felt so good taking it that she wanted to continue to support her body with it.

Mix 3 – 550 ml

Digestive Balance/Blood Sugar Support Mix: Goat's rue 50 ml, Fennel 50 ml, Gymnema 50 ml, Nettle leaf 50 ml, Black walnut 50 ml, Chamomile 50 ml, Globe artichoke 50 ml, Kelp 50 ml, Dandelion leaf 50 ml, Black cohosh 50 ml, St. Mary's thistle 50 ml.

Dose: 5 ml twice a day.

BT stayed on this mix till the end of 2012 with small adjustments here and there.

15 February 2013

Gallstones became a problem. Cholesterol went too high. For blood sugar control and liver/oils metabolism, and to dissolve gallstones, the following mix was given:

Mix 4 – 550 ml

Gallstone and Metabolic Support Mix: Calendula 20 ml, Fumitory (*Fumaria officinalis*) 20 ml, Alfalfa 40 ml, Bilberry (*Vaccinium myrtillus*) 40 ml, Blue flag (*Iris versicolor*) 30 ml, Liquorice 20 ml, Nettle leaf 40 ml, Goat's rue (*Galega officinalis*) 40 ml, Gymnema 40 ml, Black walnut (*Juglans nigra*) 30 ml, Globe artichoke 40 ml, Black cohosh (*Cimicifuga racemosa*) 40 ml, St. Mary's Thistle 40 ml, Dandelion 40 ml, Fenugreek (*Trigonella foenum-graecum*) 40 ml, Chamomile 30 ml.

Dose: 5 ml twice a day.

BT took this mix till 20 June 2013 (four months) and then did a gallbladder cleanse. Passed calcified stones in morning, and kept them in a jar to show me. They were blue crystals—big but not oily at all. May have been calcium stones.

An arthritic knee became a problem in 2010. (BT was 69.) Described as osteoarthritis with calcification seen in X-ray. We wrapped it three times a week with Carmel's oil and it got better in a few weeks. BT wrapped it regularly with this oil and managed to keep playing golf for some years.

Carmel's oil for Osteoarthritis repair – 500 ml

Include the following tinctures, do not remove the alcohol.

Ginger 10 ml, Comfrey 60 ml, Wild yam 30 ml, Turmeric/Gotu kola 20 ml, Horsetail 20 ml

Lavender essential oil 20 ml, Eucalyptus essential oil 20 ml, Rosemary essential oil 20 ml

Hypericum flowers in almond oil 300 ml

Shake well before using

This oil offers Anti-inflammatory support and Pain Relief, Joint and Bone Repair in Osteoarthritis

Apply topically regularly

At age 76 she had two knee replacements and was still managing her diet happily with no digestive difficulties or symptoms of diabetes or high BP. The only herbs she had needed were herb teas she chose for herself and occasionally taking a Respiratory Infection Mix for protection. BT had attended a course with me monthly for over two years to learn about using herb teas from the garden to maintain good health.

Some of the herbs which became important to add to BT's mixes from 2004 onwards:

Dandelion – mild herb, great tonic for liver, gall, pancreas, spleen, blood, and digestion. Tonic and diuretic for kidneys.

Globe artichoke – mild herb for upper gastric deficiency. Restores thyroid, pancreas and liver. For metabolic disorders, anaemia, hypoglycaemia.

Chamomile – aids digestion by relaxing and calming the stomach, heart, pancreas and lungs.

Ginger – to warm and restore stomach production of digestive juices, and for improving anaemia. Also helps the spleen and lungs.

Three case studies for respiratory infection treatments

Case 5

M, a woman aged 77, came in August 2006, still working full-on as a lawyer and QC—a strong and determined life force.

She told me she had been sick since February this year with bronchitis. Said she regularly gets vomiting and diarrhoea, especially after an Asian meal, and this turns to bronchial problems. If she experiences changes in climate and location, such as when travelling—she gets bronchitis straightaway—and needs to take at least two courses of antibiotics. This problem has been with her since 1982—22 years ago.

In 1982 she had a terrible gastric bug and was in and out of hospital for months, with high fevers. She was put on Vibramycin for many months and then stayed on small doses of Vibramycin for two years.

This changed her body functions totally and made her susceptible to allergies. She experimented with dietary changes, eliminated everything and slowly added things back in then—and the results seemed good.

She told me she had been on antibiotics now for six to seven years because of regular bronchitis and heart struggles. Body aches and pains in muscles and joints came back recently. Finally, one month ago M went gluten- and dairy-free—feeling very slightly better. She also started taking Ultra Probioplex one month ago—never taken before—helping now with stabilising bowels and digestive comfort. At the same time started taking ionic magnesium and chromium.

She recently went to the doctor to investigate rising acidity—an endoscopy found a loose stomach valve. She was given Losec and Nexium.

M regularly gets pain from her centre under her breasts which radiates to her shoulders and up to under the ears. During a stress test with her heart specialist she suddenly couldn't enunciate, her words were back to front in her head and coming out wrong. She said when the pain happens she has difficulty breathing and her heart rate rises. These attacks happen when she is stressed but they are happening two to three times a week now. In the middle of an attack, her BP was 80/40. At Mudgee Hospital they found nodules in the lungs with a pulmonary exam machine.

She said she is going to Italy in mid-September for a holiday and she doesn't want to take antibiotics any more. She thinks they are doing her dreadful damage. And wants my help to stop needing them. I have six weeks to get her ready for travel after years of really challenging health deterioration.

I knew I needed a mix to clean out fungus and bacterial overgrowth and to restore digestive competence and comfort, to also begin restoring her heart and liver and to support every function including immunity and lung efficiency. I needed lots of medium-strength herbs and I needed to give a high dose of the total mix. I needed to remove the alcohol and top it back up with honey so she was not ingesting a high daily intake of ethanol alcohol.

Main Mix 1 – 540 ml

Immune, Respiratory and Digestive/Liver Tonic: Rosemary, Prickly ash (*Zanthoxylum americanum*), Chamomile, Calendula, Grindelia (*Grindelia camporum*), Peppermint, Nettles, Olive leaf (*Olea europaea*), Dandelion, Parsley root, Rosehips (*Rosa canina*), Pau d'arco, Angelica (*Angelica archangelica*), Basil (*Ocimum basilicum*), Thyme (*Thymus vulgaris*), Black cohosh, Wild yam (*Dioscorea villosa*), Elderberries and Echinacea. 30 ml each. Removed alcohol.

Dose: 10 ml three times a day.

In case she got a bronchial infection while she was away I also gave her:

Respiratory and Immune Support Mix – 550 ml

Andrographis, Astragalus (*Astragulus membranaceus*), Baical/Chinese Skullcap (*Scutellaria baicalensis*), Chamomile, Lavender, Hypericum (*Hypericum perforatum*), Myrrh (*Commiphora myrrha/molmol*), Liquorice (*Glychyrriza glabra*), Mullein, Passionflower (*Passiflora incarnata*), White Horehound (*Marrubium vulgare*), Echinacea, Thyme, Ginger (*Zingiber officinale*), Elderberries, Peppermint, Ribwort. 35 ml of each herb, except Myrrh 15 ml and Ginger 10 ml, removed alcohol.

Dose 10 ml three to six times a day. To take at the same time as the Main Mix.

Supplements: Lavandula Calm – one tablet at bedtime for sleep and to take three tablets a day. Ultra Muscleze – 1 teaspoon twice a day.

Zinc Sustain – one tablet twice a day.

Oils Mix for painful shoulders, muscles, and joints—essential oils of Lavender, Rosemary and Eucalyptus (*Eucalyptus globulus*) in Hypericum oil (fresh flowers infused in almond oil).

At the end of September 2006, she came back—and had a great holiday, no antibiotics needed since starting the herbs. Dumped the Nexium and Losec. Changed diet to O blood type. No acid rising. Right now she was wheezing a bit from spring winds and builders' dust.

M thinks she can drop the long-term antibiotics if she has:

Respiratory and Immune Mix – 550 ml

As above, with Grindelia and Albizia (*Albizia lebbeck*).

Removed alcohol.

Dose: 10 ml three times a day.

I thought it a mistake not to take a repeat of Main Mix 1—I told her this.

She had repeats of this Respiratory and Immune Mix until February 2007.

M wanted to focus on her Candida overgrowth which she knew had been there since 1982. Without the Main Mix 1 her acid rising has come back depending on what she eats—sometimes she has to take Nexium.

She has pain in her stomach and chest almost all the time and gets joint pain in her knees, ankles, hips, scar tissue, and shoulders. Also has neck pain if she gets an infection, otherwise not in pain there. The stomach valve problem comes only when she has acid rising. Her bowels are a bit loose at the moment.

She went overseas in January and got a stomach bug when coming home on the plane. Needed to take antibiotics again.

Main Mix 2 – 540 ml

Anti-Candida and Gut/Liver Mix: Barberry (*Berberis vulgaris*), Greater Celandine (*Chelidonium majus*), Meadowsweet, Prickly ash, Hypericum, Echinacea, Calendula, Black walnut, Pau D'Arco, Oregano (*Origanum vulgare*), Peppermint, Dandelion. 45 ml each herb.

Dose: 4 ml twice a day.

Supplements: Kolorex caps and Ultrabiotics.

She agreed to take the Main Mix daily and keep a Respiratory and Immune Mix on the shelf to add when needed.

Phoned in for a repeat—small symptoms not noted—no antibiotics needed since going on herbs and no Nexium or Losec needed any more. She has learned which foods work for her and which don't.

Repeat Main Mix 2 – 220 ml

Replaced Barberry with Chamomile and left the rest the same as before.

In October 2008 we changed her 550 ml Respiratory and Immune Support Mix to Hawthorn berries 50 ml, Black horehound (*Ballota nigra*) 30 ml, and a bit less of all the others.

M collected and took this mix for three years. Always kept the Respiratory and Immune Mix ready to start taking but needed it less and less. Occasionally she reported in as real good or sent a message through another client in the Blue Mountains.

Case 6 (see Chapter 2, p. 11)

In February 1996, twins (D and C) were born prematurely when the mother was four months and three weeks pregnant. Both were put on a respirator and were being fed with milk powder formula.

One week into life D had pneumonia and was put on an antibiotic drip, C had bronchiolitis and her antibiotic drip had added Ventolin as well as a muscle relaxant.

One week later the twins were in terrible shape. Their grandmother arrived at my door begging me to help. She thought they would die if I didn't help with herbs.

Both were vomiting every time they were fed. C had developed a bad skin rash—more than likely an allergy to a medication. Both had been put on Phenergan, an antihistamine, which was added to their other treatments. An awful pharmaceutical overload for the twins. What options did the hospital staff have? They had no herbalist on staff.

Mix for both babies – 100 ml

Immune and Respiratory Mix: Astragalus 15 ml, Chamomile 10 ml, Liquorice 10 ml, Echinacea 20 ml, Thyme 10 ml, Mullein 10 ml, Hypericum glycerate 10 ml, St. Mary's thistle glycerate 15 ml.

Dose: 3 drops in each baby's feeding drip bottle six times a day.

Once the drips were taken away, the mother and grandmother both collaborated with dropping the doses of herbs straight into the mouths of the babies. One of them was sitting with the babies for 24 hours every day. And they knew they had to not tell the hospital staff or else they would panic because they would then be legally liable for the safety of the babies.

I wasn't removing alcohol in those days but we had glycetracts (glycerites)—it was these babies that made me start removing alcohol.

In four days D was off the ventilator and in seven days off the antibiotics—mother and grandmother had to insist on the nursing staff removing the antibiotic drips.

In ten days C was off the ventilator and the antibiotics but on corticosteroids with a Ventolin puffer handy! No more Phenergan either.

Both twins came home 3 and a half weeks after their premature birth. Their food was changed to a soy-based formula. I told the mother no wheat and no cow's milk for two years at least, maybe forever.

D had digestive sensitivities and skin rashes.

Her Mix changed to: Digestive and Skin Mix

Echinacea 15 ml, Chamomile 10 ml, Dandelion 10 ml, St. Mary's thistle 10 ml, Albizzia 10 ml. Dose: 3–5 drops in each bottle or four times a day.

C had asthma and digestive sensitivities.

Her Herbal Mix changed to: Digestive and Respiratory Mix

Grindelia 10 ml, Echinacea 15 ml, Wild cherry bark (*Prunus avium*) 10 ml, Euphorbia (*Euphorbia hirta*) 10 ml, Liquorice 10 ml.

Dose: 3–5 drops in each feeding bottle or four times a day.

The twins stayed on these mixes for over a year—with no respiratory infections and no skin problems or rashes.

Of course, the mother took them to be checked at the hospital regularly but never told them about the herbal treatment. The hospital staff and the doctors thought the twins were miracle babies. They were rung up and asked if the hospital could trial a new drug on one of the twins and the mother agreed—and the grandmother told me. I waited for the report from them. It only took a week to make the baby very sick so the trial was ended and the babes were left alone.

April 1997: 15 months old

Changed D's mix—took out the Albizzia and replaced it with a Chinese skullcap. Mix for C stayed the same. Bottle feeding stopped and we changed the dosing to 5 drops twice a day.

If either of the twins looked like they were getting an infection the recommendation was to change the dose of the mix to 8 drops six times a day until better then to drop back again.

They never got a respiratory infection, eczema outbreak or skin rash. Their mother kept them off wheat and off cow's milk products.

They stayed on these mixes for two more years until April 1999.

April 1999: 3 years and 3 months old

They stopped taking their herbs daily and just had Respiratory Infection Mix ready in the fridge containing:

Echinacea 20 ml, Grindelia 10 ml, Albizzia 10 ml, Lavender 10 ml, Chamomile 10 ml, Chinese Skullcap 10 ml, Thyme 10 ml, Liquorice 10 ml, Wild cherry bark 10 ml, Astragalus 10 ml.

Dose: 10 drops three to six times a day to fight infection.

[As described in Chapter 2, both twins went on to do great things, unhampered by their early life difficulties.]

Case 7: Dermatitis followed by bronchitis

FB, aged 57, is a smoker with high blood pressure (BP)—taking Tenormin medication. He had a bad flu this year which came back again and again. He gets patchy dermatitis, but not itchy. He wants help with the dermatitis. He is a strong fiery, funny, active golfer, a hardworking real estate agent and a loving family man.

Main Mix 1 – 110 ml

Cardiovascular/Respiratory/Skin Mix: Horsetail 5 ml, St. Mary's thistle 10 ml, Ginger 5 ml, Yellow dock 10 ml, Hawthorn 10 ml, Mistletoe 10 ml, Lime tree flowers 10 ml, Kelp 10 ml, Greater Celandine 10 ml, Rue 10 ml, Borage (*Borago officinalis*) 10 ml, Gotu kola (*Hydrocotyle asiatica*) 10 ml.

Dose: 25 drops three times a day.

18 July 1996: eight months later

So far this winter FB has had bronchitis three times. He is still coughing lots with a bit of blood in it. His cough is very dry and irritable, with only a bit of phlegm coughed up, not much, with also a sore throat and up and down glands. He has had no headaches, no nausea, or muscle aches that come and go. He feels thickly congested around the nose area and very sinusy in the head.

He is taking salmon oil, garlic, a Respiratory Infection Mix (mine), Panadol, Vit C ascorbic acid 1,000 mg a day, and Benadryl. He feels like he would be much worse if he wasn't taking my herbs. He doesn't want to take antibiotics.

I increased his dose of 1,000 mg of vitamin C to three times a day in a little water after a meal. Told him to keep taking my Respiratory Infection Mix. And made him a Main Mix as follows to repair his immune system and lungs.

Lung Repair Mix

Liquorice 10 ml, Poke root 5 ml, Kelp 5 ml, Thyme 10 ml, Chinese Skullcap 10 ml, Adhatoda (*Justicia adhatoda*) 10 ml, Marshmallow root 10 ml, Picrorhiza (*Picrorhiza kurroa*). 10 ml, Astragalus 10 ml, Wild cherry bark 10 ml, Hypericum 10 ml, Blood root (*Sanguinaria canadensis*) 10 ml.

Dose: 3 ml three times a day.

(Duplicate information above) Stay on supplements, increase Vit C to 1,000 mg three times a day.

19 August 1996: one month later

He told me his lungs feel great and he has no more infection. His head is completely clear and the mix loosened his cough and made it productive. Now he wants more of his first mix because his skin dryness and psoriasis came back bad with the flu and his first herb mix, Main Mix 1, got rid of it totally.

Repeat Main Mix 1 – given.

Then FB rang for repeat Lung Repair Mix 2—Echinacea instead of Blood root. This mix was taken as a daily mix.

He's been getting 500 ml mixes with a combination of Mix 1 and 2. This is hard—I have to work out which herbs have finished repairing and which herbs are now needed to restore his organs' functions.

18 January 2001

Phone check-in showed the changes needed—Echinacea stayed in instead of Blood root; Fennel instead of Picrorrhiza; Stoneroot instead of Poke root. His wife tells me symptoms as they come—there's a slight haemorrhoid happening!

30 August 2001

Bad bronchitis.

Bronchitis Mix – 510 ml

Astragalus 75 ml, Ribwort 45 ml, Grindelia 45 ml, Ginger 45 ml, Wild cherry 45 ml, White horehound 45 ml, Chamomile 45 ml, Lavender 45 ml, Echinacea 75 ml, Elderflower 45 ml. Dose: 3 ml twice a day for prevention and six times a day to fight infection.

Got repeats of this Bronchitis Mix for daily use until 5 December 2002—16 months. Then he got repeat mixes for using just to fight bronchitis and he says he never gets sick.

At the same time, he asked for a new Lung Repair Mix—like the first one but with high BP support for daily use.

5 December 2002

Lung Repair Mix – 520 ml

Bladderwrack 20 ml, Thyme 50 ml, Chinese skullcap 50 ml, Echinacea 50 ml, Ribwort 50 ml, Mullein 50 ml, Chamomile 50 ml, Hawthorn 50 ml, Astragalus 50 ml, Marshmallow root 50 ml, Dandelion 50 ml.

Dose: 3 ml twice a day.

This was taken until 30 January 2004—14 months when Liquorice replaced Marshmallow; White horehound replaced Dandelion.

The Bronchitis Mix was ordered regularly and kept him free of respiratory infection. No, he did not give up smoking!

On 29 March 2005 after 14 months on the last herb mixes he got pneumonia. So we changed the bronchitis mix a little—added Pleurisy root (*Asclepias tuberosa*) and Liquorice. And his PSA reading went up a bit so we added Saw palmetto (*Serenoa serrulata*) and it went down fast.

Slow tweaking along the way with these two mixes until we got to:

Bronchitis Mix – 520 ml

Pleurisy root, Chinese skullcap, Grindelia, Andrographis (*Andrographis paniculata*), Ginger 30 ml each; Myrrh, Thyme, Aniseed (*Pimpinella anisum*), Astragalus, Lavender, Echinacea, Rosemary, White horehound, 40 ml each.

Dose: 5 ml two to six times a day.

Lung and Heart Mix – 520ml

Thyme, Nettles, Olive leaf, Eucalyptus, Marshmallow, Hawthorn, Liquorice, Lime tree flowers (*Tilia* spp.), Ribwort, Chamomile, Saw palmetto, Arjuna (*Terminalia arjuna*), Black horehound, 40 ml each.

Dose: 5 ml two to three times a day.

FB remains on these two mixes, still smokes (not much I'm sure!), is 77 years old, and PSA normal.

Case 8

In 1994 FT, aged 89, came in with urination problems. He told me his urinary tract and groin felt a little irritated—he had some burning after urinating, the stream was a broken stream and he was not passing enough. Dr said his PSA was starting to go a bit high and he had a little arthritis in his hands and knees. He was not on any medication and wasn't intending to take any.

He thinks it's more like gout because the pain sometimes goes down his leg to his big toes. Sometimes he felt a little bilious. Yes, he was a bit constipated but he took ¼ teaspoon of Epsom salts in water once a day and this helped him empty his bowels once a day. In the old days, he said, he emptied his bowels two to three times a day.

He was strong like a bull. He and his wife had 12 children and he'd worked on the railways until he was 75. I used to deliver his repeat mixes on my early morning walks and he would pour me a cuppa and sit with me by the woodstove telling me stories from his life while I drank it. He stayed on the following mix for three months—within two weeks he was urinating fine with no burning. His PSA went back down and his arthritic pains went away.

Herb Mix – 110 ml

Urinary Issues and Arthritis Tonic: Buchu (*Agathosma betulina*), Red clover, Cleavers (*Galium aparine*), Yellow dock, Saw palmetto, Yarrow, Horsetail, Celery (*Apium graveolens*), Hops (*Humulus lupulus*), Hydrangea (*Hydrangea arborescens*), Marshmallow root. 10 ml of each.

Dose: 30 drops four times a day.

Reasons I used the herbs in the above mix

Buchu – soothes irritation, for inflammation and discharge in the urogenital tract.

Red clover – for clearing deep toxins, especially in the lower body, and for repairing tissue.

Cleavers – specific for non-specific urethritis (NSU), prostate, and urethra problems, inflammation in males for stones/gravel and pain on urinating.

Yellow dock – for bilious complaints and congested liver.

Saw palmetto – for atrophy of testes and for clearing growths, reducing PSA.

Yarrow – increases the ability to absorb nutrients, for restoring after a long illness.

Horsetail – strong eliminator, breaks up and removes calcium deposits, arthritis.

Celery – alkalising – for arthritis, to balance acid waste, for very white iris with calcium ring forming.

Hops – tonic and sedative as well as digestive aid. For hyper mental energy with chronic worry and insomnia.

Hydrangea – for long-term infection in kidneys and bowel, for gallstones and gravel with fluid retention. For non-specific urethritis cystitis, pyelitis.

Marshmallow root – for soothing demulcent in the intestinal and urinary tract.

I treated FT for ten years, always with these doses, and very small variations from this first mix. Also, simple tonics like Dandelion and Chamomile to restore organs and systems.

He said the mix helped him feel consistently strong and pain-free. His PSA stayed low and he remained arthritis-free and urinating easily. He eventually died of heart failure at age 99 [see Chapter 2 for details].

Case 9

JH, aged 81, date of birth 19 November 1914, came to me on 22 September 1994.

This is what she told me: 'It's my legs. It started in my toes—they were cold and numb all the time and sort of dead feeling. Could be my arteries. The doctor said it was erysipelas. He sent me for an ultrasound—that came back okay. It started in 1980 and in 1982 the doctor arranged a biopsy of a piece of calf muscle. He said they found a speck of dust. I've had regular runs of chilblains now every winter'.

In 1966 JH had nephritis and the doctors removed one kidney. She also had a hysterectomy the same year. She was on Zyloprim since then to prevent the possibility of kidney stones or as she said 'to keep acid out of her kidney'—one per day—which she doesn't always take. Also on medication for high BP which was actually sometimes high and sometimes not, and a diuretic tablet.

She had a cancer lump removed from her breast at age 78 (three years ago) and was put on daily Tamoxifen to prevent more breast cancer from developing. She said it made her feel terrible. Because of varicose veins, she had her arteries stripped from her legs eight years previously. She said her doctor had tested her circulation and said it was fine. She told me she had diverticulitis so is very careful what she eats.

I asked her if she was afraid of breast cancer developing again. She said no and that she would rather not take the Tamoxifen. She decided, without my advice, to stop taking Tamoxifen.

Herb Mix – 110 ml

Heart and Circulation Tonic: Kelp 8 ml, Hawthorn 8 ml, Bilberry 8 ml, Rue 8 ml, St Mary's thistle 8 ml, Fenugreek 8 ml, Prickly ash 8 ml, Nettle 8 ml, Jamaica dogwood (*Piscidia eurythrina*) 8 ml, Sarsparilla (*Smilax officinalis*) 8 ml, Ginkgo (*Ginkgo biloba*) 20 ml, Meadowsweet 8 ml.

Dose: 20 drops four times a day.

All the herb medicines in this mix were Nature Spirit 1:8 strength and alcohol was *not* removed. After the first bottle when I checked on JH apparently all her difficult symptoms had gone—her toes were not cold and numb any more, her digestive difficulties were better. Her erisypelas/cellulitis pain in her leg had gone.

Repeat mixes were given to JH until April 1995—12 months. Her response to the herbs was fast and good. I kept her on the same mix to establish the repair.

The reasons I used the herbs in the mix

Kelp/Bladderwrack (*Fucus vesiculosus*) – for fluid exchange, supporting thyroid and kidneys, and nourishment.

Hawthorn – heart strength and BP stabiliser.

Bilberry – nourishment and circulation, eye strength.

Rue – for veins, bowels and blood. For portal vein congestion, constipation and high BP probs as stoic people build arterial pressure and get back pressure in veins which can haemorrhage.

Dandelion – supporting and restoring liver.

Fenugreek – to help digest fats and balance the fat/water content of cells.

Prickly ash – antispasmodic and calmative for blood vessels – peripheral circulation. For leg pain, chilblains and muscular rheumatism.

Nettle – fast iron tonic, for restoring arterial circulation, especially to the brain.

Jamaica dogwood – toxic in large doses – for nervousness and insomnia, for facial and sciatic pain.

Sarsaparilla – adrenal support, alterative for blood, liver and fluid retention.

Ginkgo – circulation to the brain, inhibits platelet-clumping to help deal with side effects of pharmaceuticals, and whole body restorative.

Meadowsweet – GI normaliser with pain relief, ant-acid, many aspects of digestive assistance and oedema.

Footbath Mix—220 ml

Hypericum oil is made with fresh flowers in organic almond oil, essential oils of Lavender 10 ml and Rosemary 10 ml, and homemade Comfrey tincture 20 ml.

Dose: Add 20 ml to a bowl of hot water full enough to just cover feet. Soak your feet in this for 30 minutes after dinner and before bed three times a week.

After three months on these herbs with repeat mixes and the footbaths, JH had no pain in her feet or legs and her chilblains had disappeared. Also, her sleep was much improved and her regular gut pain was gone. She phoned me for help with a flu infection next.

    I treated JH for eight years until she was 89 and went into a retirement home. She wanted to come off all her tablets from the doctor—said they all made her feel sick. I told her not to discuss it with me but with the doctor.

    Years later she told me that what she did was tell the doctor she felt good and was happy taking herbs. While being treated by me she came off her BP tablets, her Zyloprim, and her Tamoxifen and didn't tell me for a long time. She didn't tell the doctor either and he was happy because her BP was fine. She died quite suddenly at 90 of kidney failure. Not bad for only one kidney since 1966.

    While seeing me one day she had remembered a time when she was a young woman in Sydney when she could go to her local pharmacist and get a herb mix. She told me that was always enough for her and always sorted her health problems out really well. She used to take her kids there too when they were sick. She missed the herbs and was very happy I came to live nearby.

    The doses I put her on were always 20 drops four times a day except when she got the flu—then I recommended 20 drops every two hours.

Case 10

In 1995, RC, age 18, came with her mother to see me. Her mother, a naturopath, had heard of me through a mutual friend. She said I was her last hope before they went back to the heart specialist.

The diagnosis from this heart specialist was 'supraventrical tachycardia' and 'ectopic arrhythmia'. He said she had two electrical pulses in the heart instead of one. These pulses control the heartbeat. This specialist advised mother and daughter that open heart surgery was needed to cut out one of the electrical controls and after this there would be no more tachycardia and no more emergencies.

He considered that her attacks were part of the double heartbeat pumping too much blood into her heart and that this blood spilt over into her lungs, preventing her from breathing—and so she temporarily died, drowning in her own blood during the attacks, and needed major emergency resuscitation.

I questioned this young woman closely. I felt reassured that her mother was a good naturopath and had her on all the right supplements. I just needed to diagnose her in my own way and figure out the herbs that would repair her. I agreed with her mother that the heart surgery would not help her.

Her symptoms started four years previously (she was then aged 14) with viral hepatitis and an Epstein-Barr virus at the same time. Then six months later she got a serious case of chickenpox. She had post-viral syndrome with chronic fatigue and her symptoms got worse and worse until they became life-threatening.

RC was able to describe the symptoms that warned her of the beginning of the attacks and said she has 10–20 minutes before passing out. After passing out she needed an ambulance with life support and to be admitted to the ICU where they kept her alive while they pumped the blood out of her lungs. These attacks had now become monthly and increasing. I interpreted her description of the symptoms as panic attacks. They began with breathlessness and rising from the lower belly came a wave of deep and strong anxiety. After a long discussion of her history, this was how I treated RC:

Emergency Heart Mix – 110 ml

Black horehound 10, Bugleweed (*Lycopus virginicus*) 10, Pasque flower 10, Chamomile 10, Lime tree flowers 10, Withania (*Withania somnifera*) 10,

Mistletoe (*Viscum album*) 10, Kelp 10, Motherwort 10, Black cohosh 10, Gelsemium (*Gelsemium sempervirens*) 10 drops *only*.

Dose: 30 drops four times a day.

For threatening attacks 10 drops under the tongue every 5–10 mins.

Since starting on this Emergency Heart Mix at 30 drops four times a day and her first Main Tonic Mix as below at 30 drops four times a day, RC never had another attack. But she carried the Emergency Heart Mix with her for four years and took it religiously four times a day.

Main Tonic Mix – 110 ml

Hypericum 10 ml, St. Mary's Thistle 20 ml, Fennel 10 ml, Lady's mantle 10 ml, Fenugreek 10 ml, Black Cohosh 10 ml, Elecampane 10 ml, Goat's rue (*Galega officinalis*) 10 ml, Gymnema 20 ml.

Dose: 30 drops four times a day.

This Main Tonic Mix was to be taken concurrently with the Emergency Heart Mix. With this Main Mix, over four years, we worked on restoring the functions of her body and repairing organs and systems.

At first, she had total exhaustion, lots of sugar cravings, no energy, post-exercise inertia, no menstrual cycle, and very poor ability to digest many foods with reactions and sensitivities, painful joints, difficulty sleeping, severe brain fog, and easily caught infections.

We know this condition as post-viral syndrome, more commonly known as chronic fatigue. Doctors have nothing to help—they say 'Rest' and 'Take these antibiotics' and 'It's all in your mind' and 'Go to a specialist and they will have a "simple surgical procedure"'.

Why I gave her the herbs in the Emergency Heart Mix

Black Horehound – for nausea and vomiting, nervous indigestion.

Pasque flower – for constant anxious apprehension with flooding adrenals.

Bugleweed – reduces rapid heartbeat from over-active thyroid, for internal haemorrhages of lungs.

Chamomile – relaxes the stomach and lungs, and works down the vagus nerve, for nausea with stress.

Lime flowers – for digestive support, for antispasmodic, relaxing in the upper body, anticoagulant, for nervous excitability, hysteria and insomnia, and headaches with high BP.

Withania – adaptogen for chronic fatigue syndrome (CFS) and immune support. Restores liver and digestion.

Mistletoe – for epilepsy and convulsive nervous disorders, neuralgia, delirium, hysteria, St Vitus' Dance (involuntary muscle twitching). Lessens heart reflex irritability. *Beware* of the opposite effect if too much is given.

Kelp/Bladderwrack – glandular tonic especially thyroid, whole body tonic support.

Motherwort – Nerve and heart sedative, for angina and tachycardia from hyperactive thyroid, for hypertension.

Grindelia – bronchodilator, releases lungs, symptomatic relief in asthma.

Black Cohosh – antiviral, releases muscular stress in asthma and migraines.

Gelsemium – 10 drops ONLY in this 110 ml mix—for heart oppression and constriction around the chest, for any phobias which affect heart rate.

After four years she no longer needed her herb mixes. She became a normal, healthy young woman. Strong and ready to live without her Emergency Heart Mix. She got on a plane with her friends and travelled around Europe for six months. She and her mother are still in touch every six to 12 months to assure me she still has nothing wrong. This year, 2024, she is 45 years old. She is healthy, happily married, working, and a mother of a teenage son.

CHAPTER TWENTY FIVE

Topical applications

Ever since I first experienced the herbal creams my nanna used on me I have loved the idea of applying herbs to the skin and feeling the creamy, oily, herby blend being carried inside me to work magic. Through my experience of this, I have always loved the opportunity to create a medicine blend for a patient to apply to the outside which will be absorbed through the skin and be easily available to heal something inside in need of help.

I don't like soggy parcels of hot herbs wrapped in fabric and applied to the skin. These are known as poultices. They are a traditional treatment and well known as successful over many centuries. They need to be created and applied by the herbalist as supervisor. Or at least by the user. No thanks. Much too messy.

If I was a herbalist in Europe working with the wandering armies of Alexander the Great or Napoleon's armies I would be using herbal poultices made from herbs growing around me for healing battle wounds and for fighting wound infections. That's why the skills of these medicine women were so precious to Napoleon and Alexander—they captured the most precious village healers as they travelled and forced them to follow in caravans with their tools of trade. In Alexander's time, these women were the spiritual leaders and most respected people of their tribes and villages—equal to tribal chiefs.

However, Alexander lived during the occupation of the Celtic tribes with their worship of nature and the respect and elevated social status of their Druid priests and priestesses. Roman and Christian wars hadn't started yet.

I have lived and worked as a herbalist in Australia since 1980. I have to grow my own herbs or buy medicines from manufacturers that import herbs to make my tinctures. My dispensary is made up of herbal liquid tinctures. I like to create something effective in a jar that a patient can take home and use as needed.

This means I love making special creams for healing specific conditions like bruising, varicose veins, haemorrhoids, cysts, blocked lymph glands which can lead to cysts, skin infections, bruising, blood clots near the surface of the skin, deep wounds, etc.

All my special creams were developed for a patient in need or a family member. Some difficult problems which presented to me are as follows.

Eve's blood clot

Eve came to see me about quite a large blood clot behind her knee. I had been treating her for some time and Eve had a history of liver struggles, a weakness of her liver. She wanted to know if I could help dissolve her blood clot. I didn't know the answer to that but I knew that Warfarin would poison her liver. The doctor wanted to put her on Warfarin and put her into hospital so they could make sure she would be safe if the clot started to break up and travel to somewhere dangerous.

Eve was a retired nurse and she knew that Warfarin would be very toxic for her since one of her liver problems involved not being very good at clearing blood toxicity. Which is why Eve came to me for treatment with herbs. We both knew that she needed to give Warfarin a go. So off she went to the hospital. She told the doctor she would give it three months and then she wanted to try herbal medicine to clear the clot.

The Warfarin did nothing and Eve got sicker and sicker. After three months she told the doctor she wanted to go home and she was going to take herbs. She gave him my phone number and he rang me. He asked me curtly if I knew what I was doing. And whether I knew what herbs to use.

I didn't tell him what herbs I was going to use. I never do that—I believe it is not something doctors can understand and can easily lead to misunderstandings.

I simply told him that I knew what to use to dissolve serious bruising in an old injury. And since blood clots consist of old blood coagulating in a blood vessel that had a collapsed wall, I told him I would be using my knowledge of herbs to clear out old bruising. I said that I was one of the best herbalists around and that I would be doing my best. I asked him kindly if he could be on call and available for our patient, an experienced nurse, in case she felt that an emergency was starting to happen.

He asked me to treat her from the outside only and he would then halve the dose of Warfarin and see if we could dissolve the clot with this combination of approaches. I said we could try and Eve said yes, but only one month with this approach.

I don't give amounts in this mix because it is merely an example of what can be done.

Ingredients

Dried herb tinctures of Witch hazel (*Hamamilis virginia*), Horse chestnut (*Aesculus hippocastanum*), and Arnica (*Arnica montana*).

Fresh herb tinctures of Yarrow, Lavender, Chickweed (*Stellaria media*), Mullein, Comfrey leaf, Gotu kola, Lady's mantle, Rose (*Rosa damascena*), Soapwort (*Saponaria officinalis*).

Hypericum oil—fresh flowers infused for four to six months in sweet almond oil.

Oils of Flaxseed, Wheatgerm, Sesame, and Rosehip.

Essential oils of Sage, Hyssop, Myrrh, Tea tree, Rosemary, Cypress, Lavender, Lemon.

Himalayan Flower Enhancers—Gulaga Orchid, Vital Spark, Gateway, Sludge Buster.

Instructions

Each evening put three capfuls in a shallow footbath of warm water and soak feet for 20 minutes. At bedtime apply mixture generously to a strip of cotton fabric. Wrap this around the leg where the clot is. Cover with

Glad Wrap (cling film) then a bandage. Put a covered hot water bottle next to it and leave it on for the night.

In one month this treatment had made the blood clot one third smaller. Then Eve told the doctor she wanted no more Warfarin. She wanted herbs to help her poor liver from the inside as well as herbs and oils to dissolve the clot from the outside.

It took three more months to dissolve the blood clot—with no emergencies for Eve. Her doctor saw the results. Did he ring me to say well done? *No.*

Healing scar tissue

One day I got a phone call from my friend, CN, a Chiropractic Applied Kinesiologist in Sydney. He told me that our guru of Applied Kinesiology, Dr Keith Keen (who passed away in 2021 at age 82) was finding that some women's Caesarian scars were affecting the functioning of their legs 20-plus years later. He wondered if I could make a cream to heal these scars and help reconnect damaged nerves and blood vessels.

I used the following ingredients (see below) to make the cream which was used by many women with varying degrees of improvement.

I later used this same recipe for facial scarring of the mother of one of my students who had suffered bad injuries after a car accident. My student asked me to send three jars. After using the three jars her mother said there were good changes and healing. She wanted five more jars. She used the cream for a year and sent me a special thank you with a gift from her daughter. She told me that under make-up her scars were almost unnoticeable.

Old scars hold traumatised cells in the memory of the repair tissue. I imagine Rescue Remedy or a flower essence mix that could have been applied at the time of the original trauma to support healing without locking the trauma in the cells and so blocking the best healing from happening. I imagine the emotions that may be locked inside the traumatised cells as I figure out the flower essences needed for the cream.

Healing Caesarian and perineum scars

Beeswax and shea butter

Wheatgerm oil

Flax seed oil

Rosehip oil

Fresh plant tinctures of Comfrey root, Comfrey leaf, Calendula.

Himalayan Flower Enhancers—Down to Earth for the base chakra, Wellbeing for the second chakra, Children's Flower, Vital Spark.

Bach flowers—Rescue Remedy, Star of Bethlehem.

Humanifest essences—Emerald, Moonflower, Pink Flannel Flower.

Humanifest Heart Oil.

Essential oils of Lavender, Lemon, Ylang ylang.

Pain relief oils and herbs for psoriatic arthritis (see Anita in Chapter 8, p. 51)

The oils are chosen for their ability to feed muscles, ligaments, and fluid in the joints with the ingredients needed for restoring tissue as well as carrying the herbs deep inside to help uniquely with healing the particular damage in Anita's joints.

The Hypericum oil is of course made with freshly picked flowers and some upper leaves, then blended immediately into the almond oil—and left to macerate for three to six months. Bottled and stored carefully with no air left in the top of the jar/bottle. When I press the plant matter out of the oil, the oil I get is thick and dark red—not transparent pink.

Anita's herbal oil wrap for repairing arthritic joints

Ingredients

Fresh herb tinctures of Hypericum, Comfrey root and leaf, Meadowsweet, Calendula, Lady's mantle, Gotu kola, Horsetail, and Ginger.

Hypericum oil—fresh flowers infused in sweet almond oil.

Oils of Sesame, Flax seed, Wheatgerm.

Essential oils of Rosemary and Lavender.

Himalayan Flower Enhancers—Aura Cleansing, Let Go, Vital Spark, Hidden Splendour.

Apply generously with dressings at bedtime. Wrap over the top with Gladwrap [clingfilm]. Leave on overnight.

Osteoarthritis and calcium spurs

Caroline was one of the first patients who came to see me in 1985. She brought her husband and two children—a daughter aged 11 and a son aged 8. They all came to learn how to manage their health with diet and herbs.

Caroline was my age and when we were both going through menopause she came with awful pain in her upper spine and neck which was preventing her from sleeping. After we had looked at the hormone balancing she needed help with, I made her the mix below to apply to her upper spine and neck before bed.

I told her, 'Time to go to a doctor and get an X-ray to see why this pain is here. Meanwhile, this blend will help you. Please go to the doctor real soon and let me know the results'.

She rang me three weeks later. She reported, 'The X-ray showed calcium spurs happening in three spinal joints. The doctor said it was the beginning of osteoarthritis. No treatment is available except painkillers. Don't worry though, the oil worked for me from the first application. No pain all night. I'm happy to keep applying it—I don't care if the sheets get stained'.

I planned this oil mix to be for strengthening her bones and healing any reasons for pain—inflammation, or bone spurs from thinning bones. Horsetail can dissolve bone spurs and is a great addition to any blend for healing joints and strengthening bones with its high content of silica. Mixed along with Comfrey the bones in Caroline's spine were all going to get stronger. The Wild yam was bringing anti-inflammatory action and plant progesterone and oestrogen precursors. And Ginger was bringing warmth and anti-inflammatory actions. The warmth would draw circulation and activate repair. That's what I wanted, what I imagined as I was blending it.

Three months later Caroline was forgetting to apply the oil blend every night. She only felt she needed it one or two times a week. After six months she hadn't thought to use it for a few weeks. Time for another X-ray. This one showed *no* bone spurs and stronger bones. I have since used this recipe for many people and made it my recipe for my very popular anti-inflammatory pain relief cream.

Caroline's herbal oil for osteoarthritis repair

Ingredients

Dried herb tinctures of Ginger, Wild yam, and Turmeric.

Fresh herb tinctures of Horsetail and Comfrey root.

Hypericum infused in sweet almond oil.

Essential oils of Lavender, Rosemary, and Eucalyptus.

Himalayan Flower Enhancers—Aura Clearing, Gulaga, Nirjara, Vital Spark.

Apply each night before bed.

Tom's mixes (for extensive trauma after a motorbike accident, see Chapter 4, p. 25)

When I mixed up the blends to take down from my Blue Mountains medicine garden to the huge floor of the Accident and Injury ward in the Sydney hospital, I knew that I wouldn't be able to drop herbs into Tom's mouth. And I knew it didn't matter—because everything I put on his body would go straight into his bloodstream through the skin.

Trauma: herbal oil to take the shock out of the flesh

To be applied every two hours for five days before applying the Herbal Oil Mix (below). Applied by pouring and smoothing with gentle hands—applied to every part of his body possible—poured into neck brace; poured over face; poured over bandages and into eye sockets; poured into top and bottom of leg cast and shoulder dressing. I wasn't worried about wetting him or his dressings. He was in a coma. If I got his dressings wet it meant the treatment stayed instead of being wiped off or drying up.

Trauma: Flower Essence Mix – 50 ml

Himalayan Flower Enhancers (Vital Spark, Healing, Renaissance, Gateway), 10 ml of each essence.

Australian Bush Flower Essences (Emergency Essence, Sundew, Red Lily) 2 ml of each essence.

Bach's Rescue Remedy 1 ml.

Homoeopathic liquid Arnica 1 ml.

Homoeopathic liquid Symphytum 1 ml.

Homoeopathic liquid Hypericum 1 ml.

Dose: 4–7 drops under the tongue as needed.

Topically

Humanifest oils—Heart Oil, Consecration Oil, Peace Oil—can be applied topically in times of trauma.

Herbal Oil Mix for Tom's repair

Applied every three hours after applying the flower essence mix for shock as above.

Dried plant tinctures of Arnica.

Fresh plant tinctures of Comfrey leaf, Comfrey root, Gotu kola, Calendula, Selfheal (*Prunella vulgaris*), Lady's mantle, Rose (*Rosa damascena*), Yarrow.

Hypericum fresh flowers in sweet almond oil.

Essential oils of Lavender and Rosemary.

Flower essence mix—as above for the shock treatment.

Homoeopathic liquids—Arnica, Symphytum, Hypericum.

After such an accident we have a huge amount of blood vessels that have exploded and leaked blood into connective tissue. This is what solidifies and becomes massive bruising. If left to solidify it will hold up and stagnate and prevent any healing from being able to happen. The body will struggle to survive at all because clearing this solidified blood is so hard. Tom could have remained in a coma for months or been unable to heal at all and just given up.

* * *

This book was inspired by Maurice Messegué, Juliette de Baïracli Levy, Nicholas Culpeper, Edward Bach, Dorothy Hall, my peers who so generously shared their knowledge, my mother, grandmother and great-grandmother, and the miraculous energies and synergistic possibilities of mixing plants and bodies.

With thanks to my patients, their problems, their needs and their faith in me.

BIBLIOGRAPHY

Avicenna, *The Canon of Medicine* (Place of Publication Not Identified: Publisher Not Identified, to 1799, 1700).

Amtz, William, *What the Bleep do we Know!?: Discovering the Endless Possibilities for Altering Your Everyday Reality* (Florida: Health Communications Inc, 2004).

Barnard, Julian, *A Guide to the Bach Flower Remedies* (Essex: CW Daniel and Company, 1979).

British Herbal Medicine Association, *British Herbal Pharmacopoeia* (London: BHMA, 1996).

Diamon, Harvey and Marilyn Diamond, *Fit for Life* (New York: Bantam, 2004).

Emoto, Masaru, *The Messages in Water* (London: Atria Books, 2005).

Harold, Edmund, *Crystal Healing: A Practical Guide to Healing with Quartz Crystal* (London: Harper Collins, 1990).

Hawken, Paul, *The Magic of Findhorn* (London: Harper Collins, 1975).

Holmes, Peter, *The Energetics of Western Herbal Medicine: A Materia Medica Integrating Western and Chinese Therapeutics* (London: Aeon Books, 2020).

Pert, Candace, *Molecules of Emotion: The Science behind Mind Body Medicine* (London: Simon & Schuster, 1999).

Popham, Sajah, *Evolutionary Herbalism: Science, Spirituality, and Medicine from the Heart of Nature* (Berkeley: North Atlantic Books, 2019).

Santoro, Franco, *Astroshamanism Book 1, A Journey into the Inner Universe by Franco Santoro* (Scotland: Findhorn Press, 2003).

Santoro, Franco, *Astroshamanism Book 2, The Voyage through the Zodiac* (Scotland: Findhorn Press, 2003).

Stanway, Andrew and Penny Stanway, *Pears Encyclopaedia of Child Health* (London: Pelham Books, 1980).

Whitten, Greg, *Herbal Harvest: Commercial Organic Production of Quality Dried Herbs* (Australia: Blooming Books, 2003).

RESOURCES

Bach Flower Remedies: https://www.bachflower.com/.
Himalayan Flower Enhancers: www.himalaya.com.au.
Horizon programme about Parallel Universes and Quantum Physics (aired 14th February 2002 on BBC2).

www.ingramcontent.com/pod-product-compliance
Ingram Content Group UK Ltd.
Pitfield, Milton Keynes, MK11 3LW, UK
UKHW021829310725
461421UK00007B/131